Offering Understanding and Encouragement for Caregivers

DEMENTIA

THE MONSTER WITHIN

John Herbert van Roekel

DEMENTIA
THE MONSTER WITHIN

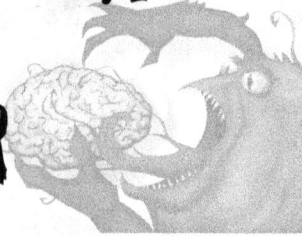

John Herbert van Roekel

Paperback Book: ISBN: 978-1-938526-48-0
E-Book (Kindle): ISBN: 978-1-938526-49-7
E-Book (ePub): ISBN: 978-1-938526-50-3

Edited and designed by Nancy E. Williams
Cover illustration by Grace Metzger Forrest

Published by SONSHINE MOUNTAIN RETREAT, INC., BLACK MOUNTAIN, NC
with the assistance of LAURUS BOOKS

Printed in the United States of America

Books may be ordered from: www.TheLaurusCompany.com/store
Electronic books are available in their respective stores: Kindle, Nook, iBooks
Also available at Amazon.com and most local bookstores.
For volume discounts, please contact: TheLaurusCo@charter.net

John H. "Herb" van Roekel is available for speaking engagements and may be
contacted at: SlayTheMonster@gmail.com

Jabberwocky

'Twas brillig, and the slithy toves
Did gyre and gimble in the wabe;
All mimsy were the borogoves,
And the mome raths outgrabe.

"Beware the Jabberwock, my son!
The jaws that bite, the claws that catch!
Beware the Jubjub bird, and shun
The frumious Bandersnatch!"

He took his vorpal sword in hand:
Long time the manxome foe he sought—
So rested he by the Tumtum tree,
And stood awhile in thought.

And, as in uffish thought he stood,
The Jabberwock, with eyes of flame,
Came whiffling through the tulgey wood,
And burbled as it came!

One, two! One, two! And through and through
The vorpal blade went snicker-snack!
He left it dead, and with its head
He went galumphing back.

"And hast thou slain the Jabberwock?
Come to my arms, my beamish boy!
O frabjous day! Callooh! Callay!"
He chortled in his joy.

'Twas brillig, and the slithy toves
Did gyre and gimble in the wabe;
All mimsy were the borogoves,
And the mome raths outgrabe.

—Lewis Carroll

(from *Through the Looking-Glass and What Alice Found There*, 1872)

Unlike Lewis Carroll's Jabberwocky, *dementia is real and all devouring to the brains and minds of its victims. We can only hope that many doctors and researchers will be able to brandish their scientific swords collectively to "slay the jabberwocky," the monster within our precious loved ones.*

Dedication

This book is dedicated to all of the families who suffer with their loved ones who are afflicted with these diseases of the brain.

We also dedicate this book to the Charlotte AFTD Caregiver Support Group. Thank you, Marlene Baker-Morgan, for your commitment to each member of our group.

I would like to give another word of appreciation to those individuals noted in the "Acknowledgements" portion of this book. My family is indebted to you beyond measure. There has been one consistent characteristic among these wonderful individuals who have been my guides. That one consistent characteristic is that no matter how brilliant or influential these leaders are, they have been remarkably kind, tender, factual, and great servants of humanity. Their kindness has been so refreshing.

You are an inspiration to all in how you make a difference in the world!

Acknowledgements

Dr. Donald Schmechle

Former Director of Joseph and Kathleen Bryan Alzheimer's Disease Research Center, Duke University Medical Center. Presently serving at The Falls Neurology & Memory Center Practice in Granite Falls, North Carolina. Dr. Schmechle diagnosed and cared for my mother-in-law, wife, and sister-in-law.

Dr. Gail V.W. Johnson

Medical Researcher at University of Rochester working on tau protein phosphorylation and function. The way she wrote her papers with such clarity inspired me to want to know more.

Dr. Kirk Wilhelmsen

Thank you for your dedication to "wanting to know" and caring for others. Dr. Wilhelmsen was the co-discoverer with Dr. Michael Hutton of the specific gene mutation R406W that is the cause of the "monster within" for my family. He also served as my daughter's genetic counselor.

Dr. Brad Boevé

My daughter's guide in discovering that there is a reason for hope. His fervor for understanding, enthusiasm to help, and encouragement is a model for the bedside manner every physician should show to the patient and caregiver.

Dr. John Hardy

Formerly, Chief of Laboratory of Neurosciences, National Institute of Aging at the National Institute of Health. This amazing leader of men showed overwhelming care in his conversations with me and directed our family to Dr. Brad Boevé at the Mayo Clinic. Thank you for spearheading a nation to confront and eventually defeat these Monsters within.

Frances Coates

Director of the Marjorie McCune Assisted Living facility, Black Mountain, NC. She and her staff embrace caring to a level that is an example for all. She truly walks beside you along the journey.

WNC Alzheimer's Association

Thank you for allowing me to volunteer. It was such a pleasure getting to meet so many who dedicate their lives to educating the community about Alzheimer's disease and other related dementias.

Project Care of North Carolina, Len Erker and his staff

Your dedication of service to families and caregivers is a model of the Christian edict, "Love your neighbor." Keep up the phenomenal job.

The Association for Frontotemporal Dementia

Your website, your mantra, and your service center are phenomenal. Keep up the great job you are doing. Thank you for the opportunities you have given me to serve.

***Planning for Hope* documentary**

Cindy Dilks and Susan Grant. Your documentary, "Planning for Hope," will be a game changer. Thank you for sharing your passion to educate others.

Fay Christine Otto

I would like to acknowledge and express my sincere gratitude to Fay Christine Otto for her vital role in gathering information for this book and helping to pull it all together. She has been an indispensable part of this project.

Table of Contents

Preface

I have written this book because there are so many caregivers who have endured years of frustration trying to get answers to their question, "What is wrong with my loved one." It is the purpose of this book to describe the dementias in simplified, general terms so that the average person can understand what has happened and what is happening to their loved one, along with a small glimpse into what might happen in the future.

After the diagnosis, caregivers have even more unanswered questions. I have deliberately presented a general approach to early-onset and late-onset Alzheimer's, Frontotemporal Lobar Dementias (Degeneration) diseases, Lewy Body Dementia, and dementias caused by trauma or other medical reasons.

This book has been written to help the caregiver understand the question, "What is causing my loved one to be the way they are?" The Alzheimer's Association and the Association for Frontotemporal Dementia provide a plethora of information. However, for many caregivers, the information is too complex. Lisa and Gary Radin have written a more encompassing text as a guide in their book, *What If It's Not Alzheimer's*.

I believe many, like me, just need to understand what is happening to their loved one. This book is a fundamental presentation of the different types of dementias together with the underlying mechanisms that contribute to their cause: brain disease caused by sick and dying neurons.

In addition, this book has a compilation of stories and perspectives written by caregivers and victims about their struggles. Caregivers endure an enormous amount of stress in providing care to their loved ones with these monstrous diseases. It helps to know you are not alone.

This book is NOT a complete guide by any means, nor is it meant to be used for medical or legal advice. It is a beginning, and it is to be used for informational purposes only. This book is only meant to be a guide, a primer if you please.

—John Herbert van Roekel

Foreword

Sharon S. Denny
The Association for Frontotemporal Dementias

We expect problems to have solutions and diseases to have cures. However, the neurodegenerative diseases broadly termed "dementias" still leave us with many unanswered questions, no effective treatments, and no cures. Dementia—the overlapping symptoms of an array of progressive brain diseases—is an unruly monster. It erodes the thinking, emotions, and awareness that make us most human. Yet, even as science pursues answers and cures, the individuals and families affected by the slow tragedy of disease point the way to the most profound human healing.

Over the past 30 years, Alzheimer's disease, the most common form of dementia, has become well recognized, with increasing research funding, medical and community resources, and public attention. There is still no treatment that stops or prevents the disease, but Alzheimer's is firmly associated with its principal symptom, memory impairment, and brings a general understanding of care needs and emotional loss. Other neuro-degenerative diseases are recognized and understood far less, even by physicians and other health professionals. A lack of awareness about the range of progressive brain disorders means people often have great difficulty getting an accurate diagnosis; families do not realize that such serious disorders can have a younger onset, and doctors don't have experience with these less common diseases.

Primary progressive aphasia, behavioral variant frontotemporal dementia, and progressive supranuclear palsy are not names that roll off the tongue easily. They are foreign terms that bring no images to mind. These are among a cluster of neurological disorders known as Frontotemporal Lobar Degeneration (FTLD). Disease in the frontal and temporal areas of the brain causes an array of progressive language, behavioral, and motor impairments. On average, FTLD generally begins in a person's late 50s, robbing them of their personality and ability to relate with others at just the point when most people are fully engaged in careers and family life. Early clinical signs of the different subtypes may be distinct, but over time they all inevitably progress to dementia, incapacity, and death.

When a clinical evaluation identifies FTLD, patients and families are frequently sent home with little or no information about what to expect. The emotional and practical aspects of providing care are huge, but the resources and support are scarce. At the Association for Frontotemporal Dementias (AFTD), we are working to change that. AFTD's mission is to promote and fund research for a future cure and to increase awareness and provide education, advocacy, and support for people affected now.

I am inspired by every person's story, especially by each patient or caregiver's unique determination to tame the monster of dementia. People confront so much over the course of the disease. They may be struggling to understand and afraid of so many uncertainties; they may be driven to learn all they can or be overwhelmed by new responsibilities to shoulder. Some people dig into the science and want to participate in research. People become persuasive advocates, finding creative ways to meet care needs against all odds. They lose sleep, money, and even friends but press on without losing heart. In time, with support and guidance, their confidence increases, and they squeeze a measure of satisfaction from doing the best they can in an all-consuming situation.

It is not at all surprising that someone confronting such a situation wrote *Dementia: The Monster Within*. Herb van Roekel exemplifies something we see often at AFTD: a passion to make the future more positive for others affected by these disorders. His family's process of discovery and contact with others struggling to understand their own situations highlighted for him the need for a readable introduction to dementias. He condenses complex information into a concise overview for the lay reader that provides a framework for understanding the science, terminology, and care planning challenges that surround the disorders that cause dementia. This book does not try to answer all the questions people may have, but it helps them to ask those questions confidently and build on a solid foundation.

The quick pace of medical research provides great hope for more accurate diagnoses and effective pharmaceutical treatments. Propelling research forward is critical, but it is not enough. We must increase awareness of neurodegenerative diseases so that when faced with changes in thinking and behavior, people can find abundant information, resources, and support. Time spent anxiously searching for a diagnosis or services cheats a patient and family of the chance to make important plans together and to live fully. Dementia gradually erodes a person over time and changes the lives of their family members forever. The future holds great promise for remarkable scientific breakthroughs. For now, we need only turn to caregivers of people with dementia who, amid so much tragic loss, teach the most important lessons of all: perseverance, compassion, and hope. ❖

You can learn more about The Association for Frontotemporal Dementias at their website: www.ftd-picks.org.

From the Heart of the Author

I am not a physician, neurologist, scientific researcher, or counselor. I am a caregiver with a science background. I have experienced almost 40 years of exposure to a specific familial form of frontotemporal lobar dementia (degeneration) called FTLD-tau (mentioned in the genetics section of The Association for Frontotemporal Dementia (AFTD) website [www.FTD-Picks.org]. The disease with which I have intimate kinship is scientifically known as R406W tauopathy. This R406W tauopathy scientific terminology is more clearly defined in the "science" section of this book (page 106). For me, it was essential to have a label for this disease. It took three decades for the medical community to give my loved one's illness a name, other than calling it "going off." "Going off" was the family's attempt to give it a name they understood.

My journey has prompted me to write this book to help you better understand that all-important question: "What is wrong with my loved one?" Most caregivers want a name to call the disease in order to feel they understand … and that they are understood. With the vast majority of these dementias, scientists have not been able to discover what causes the disease to begin.

Dementia: the Monster Within is not an extensive explanation of dementia. It is first and foremost one family's story. Our experiences may be helpful to others in recognizing signs and symptoms, the steps that are necessary to prepare yourself and your family, as well as an understanding that you are not alone. We have deliberately made every effort to keep the explanation of all aspects relating to this disease as easy to understand as possible. I have tried to employ the "KISS" system—Keep It Simple, Sonny.

At the time of this writing, I am serving as the AFTD Regional Coordinator for the South Atlantic Region of the United States. In that capacity, I have met many caregivers who simply want to understand what is happening to their loved one. The literature written by the medical and scientific community is often difficult for lay persons to understand. A fundamental vocabulary is necessary for those who do not have a scientific background yet want to understand the basics of what is happening scientifically. I have endeavored to provide that vocabulary by writing and providing excerpts directly from specific sources. The Chapter 10 "How Things Are Made" portion of this book is a "Reader's Digest" version of the science.

I experienced several "aha!" moments while surfing the web for better ways to tell this story. The first "aha!" moment was realizing **there is a knowledge revolution about dementia**. This revolution is barely 20 years old. Unfortunately, the dissemination of this information has created a paradox. The paradox is that the caregivers are frustrated with physicians for not knowing more about how to diagnose the many forms of dementia while, at the same time, physicians have a flood of information coming at them. That information, because of its newness, is constantly changing. Misdiagnoses follow more often than is acceptable, causing caregivers to be critical of medical professionals.

Many practicing neurologists are so busy taking care of their patients that the onslaught of new research information to be studied is overwhelming. It is hard to imagine the challenges they face of maintaining a medical practice, keeping up to date and informed about all of the different forms of dementia, and nurturing a family life.

Even though we grasp this, we are at times still disheartened. Let me explain why: If we go to a Psychologist with our loved one, we may receive one "diagnosis." If we go to Neurologist X, who has practiced medicine for 25 years, we may get a different diagnosis. If we go to a General Practitioner, we may receive another different diagnosis. If we go to Neurologist Y, who just graduated from 12 to 16 years post undergraduate education, we may obtain yet another diagnosis. If we go to two different major medical institutions that specialize in dementia, we may hear still a different diagnosis.

In this process of trying to find a name for the disease afflicting their loved one, the caregiver is often bewildered. They understand the importance of getting a correct diagnosis in order to give their loved one the right treatment. It is a crushing responsibility. The caregiver struggles to manage the ever-mounting responsibility of work and other parts of their intimate family relationships. This "load" can bring with it feelings of guilt as well as any number of other emotions (sadness, depression, anger, frustration, etc.).

The second "aha!" moment came when reading some of the papers on the evolution of dementias and how these diseases are grouped. **It seemed to me that there was no common denominator for grouping these diseases**.

For the sake of clarity in this book, I have categorized the dementias into two groups: "Progressive" and "Non-progressive." Progressive diseases include Alzheimer's Diseases, Lewy Body Dementia, and the FTLD sub-groups of dementias. These "progressive" diseases spread throughout the brain and are terminal. The Non-progressive group comprises approximately 20% of the total dementia cases and do not necessarily lead to death.

The third "aha!" moment was this: **The timing of when the patient is taken to the physician is extremely variable and influences the diagnosis.** One caregiver may take the patient when they first see signs of change in the loved one. Another caregiver, for a variety of reasons, may delay that first visit to the physician, psychologist, or neurologist for several years after the initial symptoms occur.

One must also factor in that the onset of most of these diseases is subtle. The "frog in the boiling pot" phenomenon sometimes applies. You can put a frog into a pot of boiling water, and he will, of course, hop out and go on his merry way. If you put a frog in cold water, however, and ever so slowly increase the heat, he will cook without ever being aware of what is happening to him. Likewise, a caregiver who sees a loved one every day can often excuse or overlook the symptoms because their onset is so gradual; whereas, an "outsider" may readily see the behavioral changes.

The behavioral changes compose part of what is a clinical history. The clinical history is vital to giving the disease a name.

How is a name for the disease obtained? Here is an analogy.

If you place six peaches out on the counter and leave them, a green mold eventually forms at a spot on the peach. Each peach may have a different location where the green spot begins, but within a couple of days, the entire peach will be engulfed as the spot spreads and gets bigger.

Let's think of that peach as the brain, with the initial site of the mold as being the starting point of the disease. We know that certain parts of the brain control various behaviors—one part controls speech, another part controls vision, other parts control cognition, anger, memory retrieval, etc. It is the initial spot, or the location of the initial damage within the brain, that determines the specific dementia name given to the disease.

The disease is "labeled" by how the patient initially responds and behaves. This behavior indicates which part of the brain is affected. Then the spot spreads to other areas of the brain, beyond its initial impact. As the disease spreads, it will progress to looking like other forms of dementia, eventually affecting all of the brain and killing the patient in the process.

Therefore, the initial diagnosis is made based on which area of the brain is first affected. If the area of speech is affected (left temporal), one name is given. If the area of executive function and reasoning is affected (the frontal lobes), another name is given. If the area of emotions is affected (lower left temporal, amygdala), yet another name is given. If the memory is affected (parietal area), it is likely to be labeled Alzheimer's disease, etc. No matter what the patient is initially diagnosed as having, all of the progressive dementias advance to look similar.

To compound the difficulty in diagnosis, it is possible that the patient may have more than one of the dementias at the same time. Is it any wonder the neurologist has difficulty correctly naming the dementia for an individual patient?

I understand the frustration of caregivers looking for answers. For me, it was important to have a legitimate name for the disease and to understand the science about the disease. Naming and understanding was not enough. I needed to have a basis for hope that an intervention or cure is forthcoming. Until recent years, there was no hope. From my perspective, there is every reason to believe that in the coming years, some of these dementia monsters will be slain.

It is my pleasure to have become friends with Cindy Dilks and Susan Grant, who have made a documentary titled "Planning For Hope." I would highly recommend that you, the reader, watch this documentary. You may order a copy at their website: www.ftdtheotherdementia.com/pre-order.html

We hope this book will create a window of hope and enlightenment that will enable readers to better understand their loved one's malady.

There Are Many Reasons For Hope

For many years I did not pursue "enlightening" others in the family about the dynamics of this disease. Families grow larger, and less intimate knowledge of individual family members ensues. Many family members had expressed that they did not want to be bothered with news that boded a horrid future for which there was NO HOPE. I did not want to alarm those extended family members I was not personally acquainted with by telling them of this disease until I had good news to share.

I reviewed the scientific literature to help me understand as much as I could about the specific dementia outlined in this book. Even though I have a science background, much of the scientific literature was well beyond my understanding. I did not relent, though, until I had a "basic" knowledge. I hope I understand enough to relate in "layman's terms" what you need to know.

There is an enormous responsibility in giving balance regarding sharing HOPE of curing these diseases. It would be incorrigible to give false hope. Yet, it is essential to give real hope.

Herein is the reality …

There is every reason to have hope. Each individual, however, needs to be realistic. Not every disease will be "cured" before causing harm to some of our loved ones. In the case of my mother-in-law, there was no hope for medical intervention. Neither is there hope for my wife and sister-in-law. Nevertheless, I have every hope for my daughter and future grandchildren.

It is a scientific fact that we are each born with somewhere between 50 and 100 billion neurons in our brains. Some use their gift of brain power better than others. It is a fact that after a few months of life, we do not grow more neurons. Once a neuron dies, it cannot be revived. Recently, scientists have given us some reasons to believe that sick neurons may be restored to better health. Conversely, when there is a brain injury, we know that, with intensive therapy, "collateral" retraining of some areas of the brain can occur. But, retraining one area of the brain to overcome injury to another area does not provide hope for the dead and dying neurons in the Dementias.

Now for the good news …

I have had the great pleasure to sit down with scientists who know the facts. Treatments and cures will come. Some scientists feel that real intervention is far into the future. Some other scientist believe that significant breakthroughs are just a few years away. Depending on the specific dementia, both groups of scientists may be correct. I believe that some treatments will be available for certain dementias very soon. Even so, it may be decades before interventions will be available for other dementias. I think this assessment is the fact and reality.

This is what I know …

There are tens of thousands of scientists in hundreds of research facilities around the world making discoveries about dementia almost daily. Some of these discoveries will lead to treatments, and some discoveries will lead to cures of some of the dementias. This enormous investment in research will pay off with dynamic discoveries.

Scientists believe the majority of dementias have either amyloid plaques and/or neurofibrillary tangles as part of the cause of the disease. A vast majority of the research is directed at understanding and finding ways to intercede in these two scientific arenas. It is only reasonable to address the largest number of dementia diseases first, then later address the more rare forms. Alzheimer's disease comprises 78% of all dementias and has both amyloid plaques and neurofibrillary tangles.

In Europe, a clinical trial for an experimental vaccine to plaque (amyloid protein) had great results. Unfortunately, the vaccine may not have been as "pure" as needed, and some deaths were reported as a result of the vaccine. The trials were terminated due to the deaths. But, investigators believe they were (are) on the right path to making a vaccine available to the general public when they make a more purified form. One must consider the wonderful history of what vaccines have done for the eradication of many diseases world wide. According to some reports, 50% of individuals who live to be 85 will develop late-onset Alzheimer's disease. Since many in our population age into their 90s and 100s, we must find a cure. I can easily believe that in the near future, everyone may chose to receive a pure vaccine to plaque, and that vaccines will block plaque formation.

I spoke with a scientist about the tauopathy associated dementias. He believes that there will be drugs available within one to three years. In fact, a clinical trial is being set up in a nearby Medical school as we write. The scientist with whom I spoke believes that within one to five years after the first drugs are released, there will be even better drugs available. He further stated that he thinks within 10 years, there is every possibility that there will be interventions that will either stop or slow the effects of the tauopathy diseases.

If we can prevent amyloid plaque and the neurofibrillary tangles from forming, we can defeat some of "the monsters within." I believe there is reason for hope! These two strategies are only two of many interventions being investigated. Truly, the "decade of the brain" has yielded hope to those of us who believe.

❖ ❖ ❖ ❖

As the research was being done for the data in this book, one thing became quite clear: the numbers cited in the literature are inconsistent. For example, one source stated that the incidences of early-onset Alzheimer's was 1%. Another source stated that early-onset Alzheimer's is 5-15%. The literature is replete with contradictions. Other sources state that vascular dementia is the second leading cause of dementia. Another source says the Lewy Body dementia is the second leading cause. And yet another source states that FTLD is the second leading cause of dementia. It is no wonder the casual reader gets confused. There is a need for more reliable epidemiology data for the range of dementias. The challenges of diagnosis and the lack of specific tests to determine clear diagnosis during life contribute to the variability in estimates of prevalence and incidence among the dementias. ❖

Introduction

Dementia ... "deprived of mind"

Dementia is a serious cognitive disorder that is due to either progressive brain disease or brain injury caused by mechanical or physiological trauma. There are actually 55 types of dementia. [More details can be found regarding Progressive and Non-Progressive Dementias on pages 21-22 and 74-76.]

Dementia results in a decline in cognitive function beyond what can be expected with normal aging. All dementias affect memory, attention, language, and problem solving at some time in the disease process. To be considered a dementia case, it is generally required that symptoms be present for at least 6 months to affirm a valid diagnosis. The progressive dementias rob the person of their mind and eventually their lives.

It is widely believed that these progressive dementias are processes of brain deterioration as a result of one or more faulty proteins or the inability of the neuronal cells to eliminate these faulty proteins. There are, as of the spring of 2009, 453 faulty genes that cause the cells to produce errant proteins that are believed to be the primary causes of dementia.

The History of Dementia

The father of medicine, Hippocrates, in 400 B.C., had the following to say on the brain disorder, epilepsy. Epilepsy is not a dementia, but I think his writing regarding the brain in "On the Sacred Disease" is relevant.

Men ought to know that from nothing else but the brain come joys, delights, laughter and sports, and sorrows, griefs, despondency, and lamentations ...

And by the same organ we become mad and delirious, and fears and terrors assail us, some by night, and some by day, and dreams and untimely wanderings, and cares that are not suitable, and ignorance of present circumstances, desuetude (inactivity), and unskillfulness. All these things we endure from the brain, when it is not healthy ... Hippocrates, 400 B.C.

Hippocrates' words ring true whether it is epilepsy or any of the dementias that affect personality and mental function. There are three other physicians who contributed to the present understanding of brain disease.

In 1801, French physician, Phillepe Pinel, described his 34-year-old patient who had lost brain function. He gave a term "demence" to describe incoherence in what he observed. The brain autopsy revealed a brain full of water and highly atrophied. From that initial French word, *demence*, the word *dementia* is derived.

In 1892, Arnold Pick observed protein tangles on autopsy of demented patients. These protein tangles were named Pick Bodies, and these bodies were noted by Alois Alzheimer a few years later. The disease that has Pick Bodies and the dementia Arnold Pick described also bares his name, Pick's Disease. This disease is among a group of diseases called Frontotemporal Lobar Dementias (FTLD).

A century after Pinel's observation, Alois Alzheimer in 1907 described his 50-year-old patient with a similar disease as Pinel's. Alzheimer had an advantage over Pinel in that he had a much improved microscope to better visualize the brain tissue. Alzheimer's basic description of the brain was the following: "... the brain being shrunken [atrophied], filled with fluid [in the ventricular spaces], damaged due to neurofibrillary tangles, and the brain tissue having bony structures [amyloid plaques]." These four characteristics are still used as the criteria to describe Alzheimer's disease. I find it ironic that both Pinel's and Alzheimer's patients fit the early-onset disease description, not the late-stage Alzheimer's, which traditionally is after the age of 65.

For the next 70 years, from 1910 to 1980, almost no remarkable progress was made in understanding brain diseases. The name given for the condition of older individuals who became demented was "senility." The medical community and society in general found it "acceptable" for old individuals to become senile (demented).

During the 1980s and 1990s, neurologists and the scientific community kept hearing of young patients with "senility," and a great deal of interest began to be focused on "what is this." This renewed interest gave rise to a decade of intense interest in neurological diseases. Because of these intense scientific investigations, the 1990s were known in the U.S. as the "Decade of the Brain" to commemorate the advances made in brain research and to promote funding for such research. Despite rapid scientific progress, much about how the brain works remains a mystery.

Since the 1990s, much has been learned about senility, dementia, and neurological diseases. Hope is beginning to shine on the 21st century for interventions or cures. Estimates suggest that 1% of the population will have a dementia by the age of 60. This number doubles every five years, reaching as much as 50% of the population over the age of 85.

Overview of the Dementias

There are 55 different types of dementia.

Of those 55, **45 are Non-progressive** dementias. They comprise approximately **20% of the cases of dementia**. These cases of dementia are **not diseases of neurons**, but **death of neurons** due to either mechanical injury or some physiological process. This group of dementias, even though incapacitating, does not generally progress to death.

Ten of the 55 different types of dementia are **Progressive dementias.** The **10 Progressive dementias** comprise approximately **80% of the cases of dementia**. Progressive dementias are caused by **diseased neurons**. They have a time of onset, and after the onset, they become worse, spreading throughout the brain until the patient expires.

The 10 Progressive dementias are listed on the next page along with a chart of the Distribution of the Progressive Dementias.

The 10 Progressive dementias include:

1. **Late-onset Alzheimer's Disease**
2. **Early-onset Alzheimer's Disease**
3. **Dementia with Lewy Bodies**

Frontotemporal Lobar Dementia (FTLD):

    4. FTLD Behavioral variant
    5. FTLD Corticobasal degeneration
    6. FTLD with Motor Neuron disease
    7. FTLD Pick's disease
    8. FTLD Progressive Aphasia
    9. FTLD Semantic dementia
    10. FTLD Progressive Supranuclear Palsy

For more about the different types of dementias, see Chapter 8: Overview of the Dementias beginning on page 73. ❖

Distribution of the Progressive Dementias

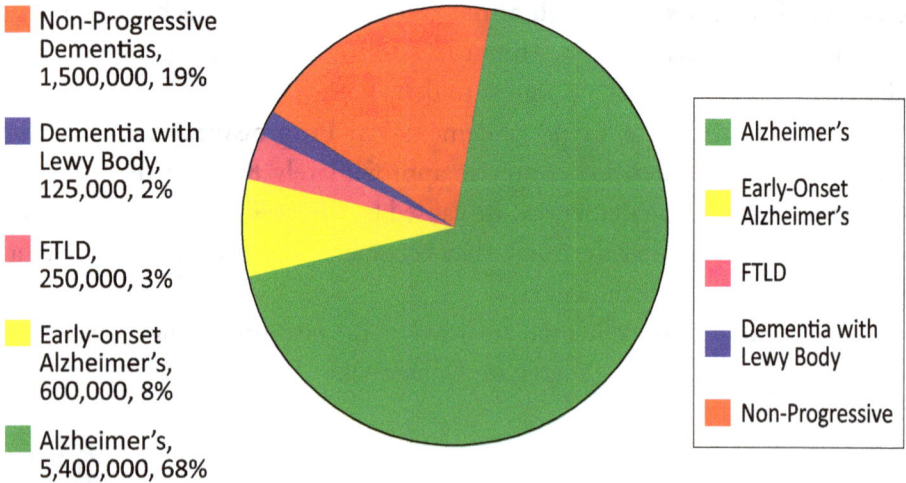

Non-Progressive Dementias, 1,500,000, 19%

Dementia with Lewy Body, 125,000, 2%

FTLD, 250,000, 3%

Early-onset Alzheimer's, 600,000, 8%

Alzheimer's, 5,400,000, 68%

Alzheimer's

Early-Onset Alzheimer's

FTLD

Dementia with Lewy Body

Non-Progressive

Chapter 1

My Story

*I*t was a balmy Sunday in November of 1965, and I had escaped the Emmanuel College church patrol again. Emmanuel College was in the heart of Northeast Georgia, four hundred miles from my home in Wilson, North Carolina.

It was a requirement of the college that all students attend church every Sunday morning, but as a cafeteria worker, I somehow eluded "the patrol" to get my Sunday morning nap. By lunch time, I was at my post behind the window where all the trays were brought at the end of the meal. Most often, I was at my post as the lines of students and visitors came through the lunch line. This was my opportunity to scope out the prospects of the young damsels preparing to get their meals.

On this particular Sunday morning, Carol Stevens had her attractive younger (by two years) sister, Evelyn, visiting from North Carolina. Evelyn was a nursing student at North Carolina Baptist Hospital in Winston Salem. She was tall, curvaceous, and appeared to be intellectually stimulating. My first impression was that she could absolutely be considered a prospect for a relationship. I did not, however, believe I had made a lasting impression on her. Who would ever have thought our paths would cross again years later?

I left Emmanuel College after the first year because I had found my niche in the academic world. Unlike Carol, I was not a scholar, and as many freshmen do, only learned to learn during my first year of college. What I learned was that Science was my niche. Ironically, it was the very thing I avoided in high school because of my fear of failure.

I found myself walking four blocks to school at Atlantic Christian College instead of being 400 miles away in Georgia. For the next two years, I prepared myself for some kind of Science career. Midway through my junior year, I went to my academic counselor, Dr. J. P. Tyndall, and expressed to him my acute concern about having no direction for my life. "Dr. Tyndall, what am I going to do?" After some discussion, he asked me what I did not want to do. I expressed my disdain for any type of sales or automotive career. He suggested that I was probably a "service" kind of guy (service personality) and suggested that I should explore the field of Medical Technology.

Since I knew nothing about what a Medical Technologist (Lab Technologist) does, he recommended that I go to Wilson Memorial Hospital and speak with Tony Christiano, the Chief Laboratory Technologist/Laboratory Manager. I have no recollection of what Tony told me or showed me that day, but I do recall the absolute enthusiasm he had for what he did. His job must have been fantastic for him to enjoy his career that much. That was the kind of career I wanted as well. So, a path was chosen.

Atlantic Christian College had an affiliation agreement with Wake Forest University through the NC Baptist Hospital Medical Technology Program. As such, I would be completing a 3/1 program—three years in the Academic Scholastic Program and one year in the Intern program at NC Baptist Hospital in the field of Medical Technology. Thus, at the end of my one year, I would receive a diploma from Atlantic Christian College with a bachelor of science degree and a Certificate of Completion from NC Baptist Hospital and the affiliate, Wake Forest University. Upon receiving the BS in Science, I would take the National Registry as a Medical Technologist, certified by the American Society of Clinical Pathologists (ASCP). This I did.

Being that I am six foot three and 220 pounds, I found myself delighted to be standing in the hospital cafeteria lunch line often. One Tuesday morning as I was doing just that, to my surprise an attractive, tall, curvaceous nursing student asked me, "Are you Herb? Did you attend Emmanuel College?" Evelyn confessed later that she had to borrow money from a friend so that she was able to get in line behind me. It was all a strategy. Apparently, I had made some kind of impression two years earlier after all. To be honest, at first I did not recognize her as someone I knew until she explained that she was Carol Stevens' sister. Who would have guessed that a second meeting would lead to a hot and steamy relationship where I, the pursuer, was in hot pursuit?

Evelyn would be finishing her three-year nursing program approximately nine months after my program was complete. She decided to stay employed there in the nursing field, and I was the first male to be employed in the Chemistry Laboratory. I was starting at the bottom rung. (I could have gone to work in the Blood Bank, Hematology, Urinalysis, or Microbiology sections, all of which comprise the total field of Medical Technology.)

After a romantic courtship, Evelyn and I married on October 17, 1970. For the next eleven years, I would hear conversations among the family about someone "going off" and having to be placed in some kind of institution. There was never any explanation of what was truly meant by "going off."

In those eleven years, I went to Broughton Hospital and met Evelyn's grandmother from the maternal side of the family. Evelyn's grandmother was Ethel Plem. She was in her mid to late 70s. She simply sat in her chair, had a far off look, a childish grin, and only responded to stimuli, not knowing who she was responding to. This gave me a preview and understanding of what "going off" meant. I remember thinking, what the heck have I gotten myself into? I found out later that Ethel Plem's brother, Albert, was in the same facility with the same malady. Neither of them recognized anyone as an intimate family member. (Their behavior was similar to that of Terri Schiavo, the woman in the Florida lawsuit case regarding permission to withdraw life support.) Little did I know or understand that a "monster" was lurking around the corner, waiting to attack my family. I did not comprehend the darkness of the path before us.

It appears that five of the six siblings of Ethel Plem, including her, "went off" in this manner.

On the next page is a pedigree of the family. A "pedigree" is a picture diagram to express the occurrence of something being examined about a family. ❖

PEDIGREE of a Family with R406W Tauopathy

A clear circle represents a woman who does not have the disease. A pink circle represents a woman who has the disease. A blue circle represents a woman who might have the disease. Squares represents men with the same characteristics.

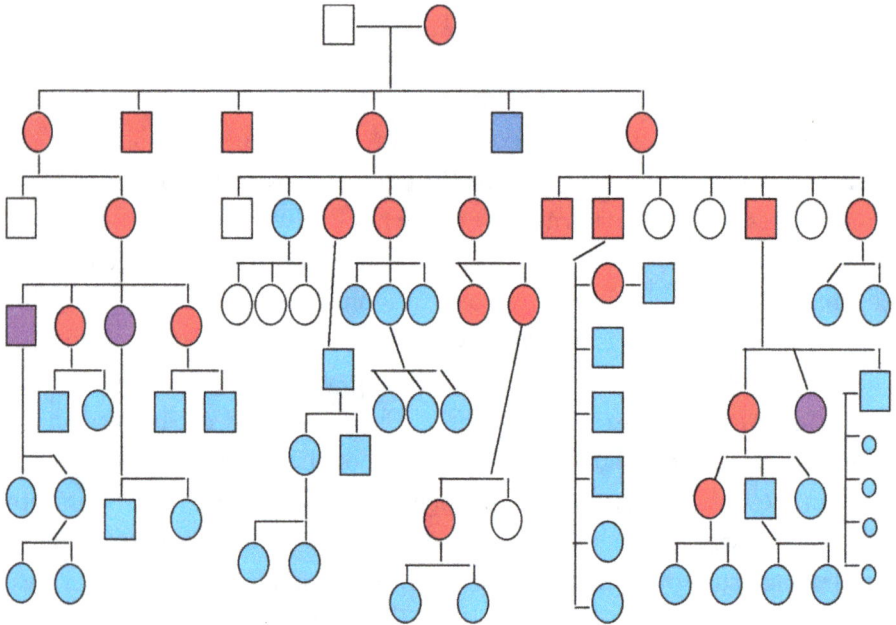

Legend

Circle = Woman

Square = Man

White = Negative

Red = Positive

Blue = Unknown

Purple = Suspected+

There may be at least 20 to 30 other blue circles and squares (unknown) that could be added to this pedigree, for whom we were unable to get information. These, plus the ones pictured above, represent approximately 25 cases (if we assume the 50/50 probability of genetic inheritance). See page 98 for further discussion of Autosomal Dominant Genes.

Chapter 2

Generational Afflictions

We later discovered more facts about Evelyn's grandmother. Ethel Plem was a daughter of Louisa Betterly. Ethel started becoming ill in her late 40s. She was a model grandmother—loving, caring, and tender. She would do all things necessary to keep the family happy.

Evelyn told me of the tender moments when she and Carol would be dropped off at Granny Plem's homeplace after school to wait for their parents to pick them up after work. She spoke fondly of those times when their grandmother would put potatoes in the ashes of the fireplace to cook. They were ready for the eating when the school bus dropped them off.

Carol and Evelyn once took me to the old home place with its huge rock mantel above the fireplace. There they shared their fond memories. We also went to the barn where the last of her possessions were stored, including a peddle pump organ.

One particular point of note was this. The family had to give the home place, the land, and all of the valuables to the State of North Carolina to make it possible for Ethel to be taken care of at the Broughton State Hospital. The State could not do anything with the property until she expired. For almost 30 years, the home place sat there rotting. The State then auctioned the ruined home place and property to the highest bidder. The family lost everything to this disease: their loved one and all the possessions.

As science would finally tell us, Louisa Betterly had passed down a gene on chromosome 17 not only to Ethel, but to at least four of her other children. (Refer to the science information provided on pages 73 and 106.)

This gene is a heterozygous dominant gene, which means that if one receives one copy of the gene, they will manifest the disease. There is a 50-50 chance that any child of a parent with this heterozygous dominant gene will inherit the disease. For this family, "going off" meant losing the capacity to perform daily tasks and forgetting their interactions within minutes of things happening. Also, in the later stages, they lose all of their memories and their ability to perform any and all activities of daily living (ADL).

This disease was originally called Frontotemporal Parkinsonian Dementia-17. It was later changed to Frontotemporal Lobar Dementia-17 (FTLD-17). The 17 means that it is a fault on chromosome 17. This chromosome does not have anything to do with physical or sexual presentation. One cannot look at a person and say they are predisposed to the disease or that their sex would predispose them to it.

Scientists have now discovered the actual gene flaw. It is called an "R406W gene mutation," a "Tauopathy." A Tauopathy is a genetic flaw in making a protein in the brain called "Tau." This error causes the production of neurofibrillary tangles that, over time, kill the neurons in the brain. In doing so, the person become senile, or demented. They "go off." And truly, they do "go off" to become someone who is unrecognizable. Who they once were no longer exists.

This disease, FTLD-17 tauopathy, was not discovered (named) until the late 1980s and1990s. Until then, it was simply labeled "senility," as were a host of dementia diseases. FTLD-17 is just one of the diseases under the umbrella of Frontotemporal Lobar Dementia (Degeneration)-Picks Disease. In that group, there is a subtype known commonly as Pick's Disease that is an individual disease in and of itself. There are, to this date, 453 gene mutations that cause a variety of dementias (refer to page 106). ❖

Chapter 3

Our Family

*P*rior to our honeymoon, Evelyn and I had decided to settle in the center of the state, equal distances from my family in the eastern part of North Carolina (Wilson/Goldsboro) and from her family in the mountains of western North Carolina (Asheville/Black Mountain). Evelyn was a floor nurse, and I was a bench (entry level position) chemist in the Laboratory at the same hospital. On the weekends, I worked in the Blood Bank Department of the Laboratory preparing blood for emergencies and pre-ops for Monday surgeries.

We lived at 2255 Elizabeth Avenue (just blocks from the Hospital) in a rented, fully-furnished, five bedroom, two-story house for $90 a month from October 1970 to February 1971. We rented the house from Mrs. Woodrow, who lived most of the year in Florida.

In February of 1971, I assumed an Assistant Supervisory position in Chemistry at High Point Memorial Hospital, about 30 miles away. Evelyn took her first position as a Public Health Nurse and was responsible for the care and investigation of concerns for an assigned area. Her territory turned out to be where the "Black Panther" revolutionary group resided in High Point. I could never determine whether it was her bravery or her naivety that kept her from being fearful of going there alone. It was unsafe for this attractive woman to go where a sane woman had not gone before. God truly protected her. Years later, she revealed to me that one day while going to her job, she found herself in an extremely threatening situation where she said it was as if an angel intervened on her behalf to protect her. She must have known that if I had been informed at the time, I would have insisted that she discontinue the dangerous part of her work.

Not long after that, an opportunity presented itself for an upwardly mobile change of my career. On May 31, 1972, Evelyn and I packed our bags and all of our belongings into one small U-Haul truck and moved to Siler City. We would make Siler City our home and raise our family there for the next 27 years. On June 21, three weeks to the day after we had settled in Siler City, we were saddened to learn that Evelyn's dad, Rodney, had passed away (post-operatively) at Pardee Memorial Hospital in Hendersonville, North Carolina, just east of Asheville.

Evelyn's mom, Doris, was left a widow at age 46. Rodney was 23 years older than Doris. Like other families who have lost a loved one, it was a dark time for our family, but nothing as foreboding as what was yet to come.

For the next 18 years, Doris lived alone, deep in the desolate mountains of North Carolina. We were not fully aware of the changes that were taking place in Doris and her behavior. Changes in behavior due to most dementias come subtly. Only years later did neighbors and friends tell us of her aberrant behavior, such as walking down the highway playing her guitar in her bathrobe. We also were told years later of her killing the neighbor's dog with a sling blade. She never did like dogs all that much.

Rodney, Doris' husband, had not been well since his 59th birthday when he had a massive heart attack. Since that time, he was unable to work a full-time job. Rodney was the school bus driver for the children in the neighborhood and built some furniture and church pews in his woodworking shop. He did the best he could.

Doris became the breadwinner of the family as she was so much younger than Rodney. She not only went out and made a living for the family, she looked after the family by canning, house cleaning, church work, etc. She was a typical superwoman, like so many women today. When we visited, she always had a fantastic meal on the table, and the house was neat and clean. She was hard working, competent, and a definite type A personality. All was going well for Doris until she turned 50 and the Monster came.

During one of our visits, I remember Doris saying that at times she felt like the front of her brain was frying. She would pull at her hair in frustration, as if she were going to pull it out. In hindsight, it was a significant expression, prophetic of the encroaching Monster.

For the next 21 years (1972-1993), we witnessed a continuing gradual and subtle metamorphosis. Doris, a dynamic individual who worked adeptly at a job, managed a home, was an advocate for the community and the church, became a person who merely walked around the yard and picked up sticks and leaves. She remained very interactive and expressive, but she started not being Doris. The Doris we knew and loved was slowly "going away"— another family member lost to the Monster.

Irrationally and unexpectedly, Doris resigned her job as a data punch operator. She was frustrated that she could no longer remember how to operate her machinery and learn new procedures. To show further illogical behavior and adding to our load, she absolutely refused to take her retirement entitlement from the company. From 1975 to 1990, we not only were responsible for her safety from 150 miles away, but we were also financially responsible for all of her expenses.

During this period of time, she lost all of her skills of keeping a neat house and preparing great meals, and her short term memory evaporated. My how I have missed those great meals that she prepared and those family times at the table together.

Incongruously, she learned to play the guitar and wrote songs after the manifestation of the disease. We had never heard her play the guitar prior to this time, so we assume it was a newly developed skill. She had been a piano player and singer, and even as this nefarious disease claimed more and more of her, she delighted to sit at the piano and play robustly those hymns and songs of old. I still find it so incredible that she could sing, play piano, and interact with people simultaneously right up until the disease took her life. Yet, she had forgotten her sisters and her grandchildren's names. Since Evelyn and I both worked in health care, we knew from her unique symptoms that she did not have Alzheimer's, but we were baffled at what she did have, what was making her "go off." She just did not behave like any Alzheimer's patients we had observed. (Alzheimer's was the only disease reference we had. Years later, science was to change our understanding.)

In the late 1980s, I specifically remember the frustration Doris had with the heating system in her house. It was a water-jacketed, thermal conducted system to all rooms of the house. Doris, being a fiscally responsible person, was always turning the system off, thinking she would be saving fuel. But, by turning the system off, she compromised the gaskets within the system and caused it to leak water significantly. Her short term memory was all but gone at that time, so she would call Carol, her other daughter, 25 to 30 times a day complaining about the leaking heating system. Carol was 120 miles away trying to fulfill her role as a college professor. How frustrated and hurt Carol became that she could not make her mom remember.

One of the dynamics of the human personality is the desire to feel needed. To fulfill that desire, Doris collected leaves and limbs from all over the three-acre yard and placed them in plastic bags. When we arrived from Siler City, we would find the entire back porch (6 x 25 feet) covered in bags of leaves and limbs, sometimes up to 40 bags. This was her way of showing us her productivity and how hard she had been working. It was something she could do competently, and she took pride in doing it.

Another characteristic of people with FTLD and other dementias is that they have a tendency to hoard. They are fearful that they will run out of certain commodities that are important to them. Doris' important things were paper and plastic bags, dish washing detergent, paper towels, toilet paper, and Chunky Soup. She had copious volumes of these items, enough to last ten years. We think she simply forgot that she had bought them.

Another preservation behavior is that they eat the same foods over and over. One of the rationales of this is that they can no longer comprehend how to prepare complex meals. Her three foods were Fruit Loops, Chunky Soup, and ice cream. We surmise that she chose these three things because they required no cognitive planning process.

We saw also during this period of time an erosion of her ability to make rational decisions. She became very naive and was easily led. Salesmen could come to the door and sell her anything. They could easily take advantage because she became as naive as a child.

Toward the end of this time, she loaded the wood stove in her bedroom full to the brim with wood, soaked it in kerosene and lit it. She was unable to rationalize or process the danger that she had created. Needless to say, it could have burned the house down with her in it.

The final straw that told us she could no longer take care of herself and that we had to do something was when a social worker visited and found all four burners of the electric stove lit and tea towels hung over the burners in an effort to dry the towels.

WHAT DOES ONE DO?

Fortunately for us, Evelyn had worked several years as a public health nurse, an administrative nurse at our local hospital, and the activities/admissions nurse at the local nursing home. There, she received phenomenal advice from the Nursing Home Administrator, John Ranford, on how to proceed with this tragic family crisis.

John Ranford guided us in understanding the Medicaid regulations so that Carol, Evelyn, and I would not have to assume the enormous cost of convalescent care for Doris in the nursing home. Basically, what John told us was that we had to liquidate all of Doris' assets down to $1500. We dispersed her assets as the law permitted. Monies were dispersed in accordance with the appropriate regulations at that time. (Each State may have different regulations, and as an informed caregiver, you should make yourself fully aware of these regulations well before there is a demonstrated need for these services.)

At that time, we were not aware of Home Care, Assisted Living, and Day Care for the Elderly. Since we were 150 miles away, we could not have managed those kinds of arrangements for her anyway.

It was evident by Doris' atypical behaviors that she needed constant attention. We were not able to provide this kind of attention because of her remote location nine miles into the mountainous countryside. Like many people today who are experiencing the "sandwich" generation, we had our families and careers to attend to. We could not supervise Doris 24 hour a day. In today's health care climate, there are many more options for those who are not ready for convalescent care, i.e., Adult Day Care, Assisted Living, and a variety of other combined choices. (Read more about this on page 114.)

One of the major concerns for any family member is to prepare ahead by procuring long-term care insurance BEFORE there is a diagnosis of FTLD or other serious illness. (See Chapter 11 (page 111) for what a long-term care insurance policy should contain.)

It is noteworthy to understand that with some FTLDs, it can be a 20 to 30 year process of decline. It is financially essential to have a well-written Long Term Care (LTC) policy to protect the financial assets of the caregivers and the victims of this disease. In addition, the caregivers need to apply for Social Security Disability for the victim. Social Security Disability also assists victims in being awarded Medicare Parts A and B for their basic medical needs. (Contact the Social Security Administration for more information.)

THE PROCESS OF CARING FOR DORIS

One must keep in context that the late 1980s was the time period when scientists began to differentiate these diseases from Alzheimer's and Early Onset Alzheimer's. For us as a family, we knew something was wrong but just did not know what it was. Doris was too young to be having Alzheimer's, and her behavior was significantly different from that of classic Alzheimer's.

Doris was extremely intelligent and cognitive, but she could not remember what had happened moments before. She was socially interactive, and her outspoken nature masked what is typically seen as the disinhibited behavior of this subtype of FTLD. Her intellect, her ability to learn to play the guitar and write songs, and her interacting while playing the piano were certainly not typical of Alzheimer's patients. Her personality shifts, her irrational thinking, anxiety, inability to process complicated thought, and hoarding were characteristics we did not understand, and we assuredly did not know how to cope with them.

Our inability to cope with or understand what was happening to Doris prompted us to seek medical help. One of the crucial decisions we made was to bring her to meet our general practitioner in Siler City, Dr. Brad Hausman. After his evaluation and the laboratory tests were compiled and evaluated, he recommended that she be seen by a Neurologist at Duke University Medical Center Memory Loss Clinic. Her physician there was Dr. Donald Schmechle. After many more tests— MRI, PET Scans, thyroid function, etc.—he made a clinical diagnosis that she had an "unusual form of Alzheimer's." This was very early in the understanding of these dementia diseases.

As part of this process and ongoing investigations, the family decided to enroll Doris in the post-disease diagnosis program; her brain would be donated for research upon her death. Most FTLD diagnoses can be definitely confirmed only on examination of the brain tissue after death, with some exceptions. One of these exceptions is if there is a pattern of family inheritance and an identified gene mutation for which a specific test has been developed, i.e., R406W Tau mutation. In the case of our family, this test had not been developed or was unavailable at that time.

At this point in our collective frustrations and all that goes with it, the family decided that Doris should be placed in an environment where she would be safe and could receive the care that she needed. The next challenge was how to implement the decision.

We invited her to come to visit us. We picked her up in the mountains and brought her to Siler City because we had removed her privilege of driving several months prior. One of the important vestiges of autonomy is the privilege of driving. When is it appropriate to remove that privilege? It is not an easy task to determine, but when the safety of the public becomes a greater concern than the need of the patient to have autonomy, it is time. It is not like you wake up one day and know that this has happened. Consultation with the Neurologist, your Insurance Agent, the Department of Motor Vehicles, and other family members is essential. Sometimes it is necessary to take action for the safety of all. That may require that you solicit the Motor Vehicle Department to intervene by requiring the "patient" to come in to be reevaluated to ensure they still meet the State driving standards.

Doris spent the weekend with us in Siler City. Their trait of becoming naive and easily led becomes a blessing at these times. Another blessing is that they do not remember what we would feel to be egregious actions, such as removing driving privileges. In this case, Doris became very naive and did not remember actions being taken from her that might cause hostility. Every FTLD patient is different, and your loved one may behave in a different way than the way our Doris behaved. Some do become hostile, angry, violent, and paranoid, with marked personality dysfunction.

On Monday morning following the weekend visit, I was assigned the task of taking Doris to the nursing home and leaving her there. It just happened that the nursing home that John Ranford was temporarily assigned to at that time was in Wilson, North Carolina, where my mom and dad lived. John Ranford was the nursing home administrator who had advised us on Medicaid regulations.

I asked Doris to put her luggage in the car. I told her we would be visiting customers along the way, and we might spend the night. As we approached Wilson, I was going to stop off to see one of my friends at the nursing home, and I wanted her to meet him as well.

When we arrived at the nursing home, Doris and I went in and met with John. John had his head nurse take her by the hand to have a tour of the facility, and John told me to leave. He would take care of everything else.

Some readers may see this as being cruel, insensitive, and deceptive. The truth is that this disease creates a situation where reasoning with them is near impossible and only creates anger, hostility, and fear for them.

Doris was a very physically healthy specimen, and we honestly thought that by 10 o'clock that night the nursing home would have had to put cow kickers on her and would be calling us to bring her home. The reality was, we never heard a word. She adapted quickly and easily to the new environment. We could finally rest after years of worry over her safety.

After several years at the Bryon Center in Wilson, John was able to place Doris in a unit for Alzheimer's patients in Durham, North Carolina, that was specially designed for Alzheimer's and Cognitively Impaired patients. Even though Doris did not appear or behave as other Alzheimer's patients, this was still the best fit for her at the time. Since Durham is within an hour's drive of Siler City where we lived, we were able to visit her often in her last years. Two weeks before Doris passed away in August of 1994, we visited with her. It was amazing. She could play any number of songs on the piano from memory, sing the words to the songs from memory, and interact with those around her, all simultaneously, but she could not remember the names of my children or those of her sisters when they visited. The mind is a very complex and miraculous organ. Two weeks later, she had a deep cerebral vascular hemorrhage that partially paralyzed her on her right side.

When we visited her in the hospital, she did the most audacious thing that I could ever have imagined she could do. As I leaned over to kiss her goodbye on the forehead, she grabbed me with her left arm, pulled me toward her, and kissed me right on the lips with a glowing grin on her face. It was completely out of character!

The night before she was to be discharged from the hospital to go back to the nursing home, she had an additional stroke and passed away in her sleep.

Doris' brain was donated to the Joseph and Kathleen Bryan Research Facility at Duke University. A subsequent autopsy report was sent to us stating that Doris had an "unusual form of Alzheimer's," with neurofibrillary tangles only and no plague. This is a classic description for this Tauopathy. The Monster had taken another victim from this family … how many more would be taken this way?

Thus, closure came to this portion of the dark path this family has trodden for generations. At least some light of understanding was beginning to shine upon this monstrous disease.

Once we knew the diagnosis that had been made on Doris, we knew to go back and investigate past members (ancestors) of the family. We had been told by Duke that there was no hope for the patients of this disease. As we gathered the information, we did not want to needlessly alarm family members.

As we looked back at the family of Doris' mother, Ethel, we knew that her brother, Adam, had been in Broughton with a similar diagnosis. We were told that Edward, another brother, had died of Alzheimer's, but could this also have been the same disease? We knew that Donald had never been "right," nor had his son. Donald's son had no offspring to follow the lineage. The other two brothers had no offspring, so there were no descendants there to follow to see if they had the disease.

We knew Emily Lex-Betterly had married an Edwards. This family, however, was very reticent to share or accept information regarding this disease. We knew that Zena Bell did not live long enough to demonstrate the disease, but she had a daughter, Violet, who had the disease. Violet had major personality changes and was described as being violent. Violet's daughter, Sally Ann, definitely had the disease. Janice, her other daughter, most likely did as well. There is some question about the remaining daughter and son.

That brings us to Ethel and her four children. Without a doubt, Doris, Ella Jean, and Candice all had the disease. The only brother did not appear to have shown any signs of the disease but died at 57 from a massive heart attack. One of the defining characteristics is that this specific genetic variant of the disease begins to manifest itself in subtle ways between the ages of 48 and 52.

Out of respect for the Edwards side of the family, we will not discuss the details, but we can say with conviction that of the seven family siblings from Emily Lex, at least three brothers and one sister manifested the disease, and there have been family members subsequently who have manifested it as well.

After discovering the information about the rest of the family, we were put on notice to be observant of any characteristic changes in Evelyn, my wife, and Carol, her sister.

It was at this point that we sought professional guidance in preparing the following documents: Long Term Care Insurance, a Will, Power of Attorney —Health and Financial, and a Living Health Care Will. (Samples of some of these documents are in the Appendix.) These documents are necessary for any caregiver to have for the victims of cognitively impaired diseases, whether they are Alzheimer's or FTLD. ❖

Chapter 4

Carol's Journey

*I*f there was one word to describe Carol from early childhood to the present, that word would be "exceptional." One of the characteristics of this family that has been noted is that they were and are extremely bright, and of course, some are brighter than others. Carol was the brightest of the bright, probably a genius level IQ. She graduated valedictorian of her high school class. She was top of her class in junior college. She earned a four-year bachelor of science degree at Appalachian State University and was in a graduate degree program at Wake Forest University in English Literature. She served as a college professor in English Literature for 23 years, holding many prestigious job roles. She was the first deaconess of her local church. She was well respected for her sensitivity, communication, and intellectual prowess.

Thank goodness for good friends. Carol's best friend, Terri, had experienced difficulty years before when trying to place her mother in a convalescent home. She encouraged Carol, as a result of her experience, to obtain long term care insurance and to buy an independent policy as well through Emmanuel College where she worked.

One evening years later when Carol was about 50, I received a phone call from Terri. Her best friend simply said, "What is wrong with Carol? She simply is not acting like herself anymore."

As time went by, Carol was unable to take care of her financial affairs and turned them over to me. The college, as well, kept modifying her role as esteemed faculty member down to jobs with less and less responsibility until, finally, she was simply a personal guidance counselor.

She would start teaching a subject and, midway through, forget where she was and unknowingly repeat everything from the top of the lesson. The students recognized her inability and related it to the administration. Eventually, her contract was not renewed, for she could not function at the level needed for her students to receive the education they deserved. The college was extremely good to her, allowing her to remain in her apartment on campus for a year after she stopped teaching, at no expense to her.

Carol became a prisoner in her own apartment. This dedicated educator with a brilliant mind had a Monster slowly eating away all that she was. She became extremely frustrated and angry because she did not understand why she was no longer able to teach. With Alzheimer's Disease, the patient usually senses that something is wrong. With FTLDs, they most often do not know they have a difficulty and, in some cases, can become angered that someone insinuates they do.

There she was in her apartment, wanting to teach, not knowing that she could not teach at her previous level, totally frustrated that no one would let her. Anger ... anger ... anger. Frustration ... frustration ... frustration. Her anger and frustration resulted in her alienating all of her friends. They would ask, "What has happened to Carol? The Carol we have always loved and respected has 'gone away'."

She literally had thousands of Post-It notes to remind her of what she was supposed to be doing. Her short-term memory was quickly being eroded. Her ability to do the activities of daily living continued to decline.

During that time, my youngest daughter, Anne, was sharing apartment space with her while attending the college. Anne told me that Carol was "going off." Carol's personality distortions precluded them having a viable personable interaction. One evening when Carol and I had one of our normal conversations (for us that was an animated debate), she could no longer formulate a debating strategy, and I knew that something was severely wrong.

What to do? I was not her husband, I was just her brother-in-law. What should I do with this intelligent woman who was "going off" ... what to do about Carol.

I had to make numerous visits to Georgia to remedy some of the situations Carol was creating for herself. She could not manage her finances. She was bouncing checks, going on buying sprees, overriding church policy as a deaconess, getting lost, etc. Then there was the issue of her driving privilege. She was alone there and needed a means of transportation as her knees were bad, and she was isolated at the college facility.

Terri became my greatest ally. She took Carol to her General Practitioner. Then she took her to a physician in a neighboring town for neurological/ psychological evaluation. There, she was diagnosed as "most likely" having dementia. Upon receiving that diagnosis, Terri assisted Carol in getting Social Security Disability. Throughout this process, Carol assailed and railed against her best friend. Terri endured a lot for the sake of her friend.

It is at this point that the stories of Carol and her sister—my wife, Evelyn—merge. But let me first tell you Evelyn's story. ❖

Chapter 5

Evelyn's Journey

*E*velyn was a bright, articulate woman with the ability to work within organizations. As a professional, Evelyn had many different roles and accomplishments. She had served two counties as a Public Health Nurse. She did a position paper and presented it at a major forum in Chicago having to do with the positive benefits of multi-phasic screening in a rural industrial area. She was chosen to the board of the Joint Orange-Chatham County Action Committee to promote improved rural opportunities in Chatham County. She did the administrative groundwork for establishing Hospice in Chatham County. Evelyn served the hospital as Position Service Reviewer, did Admission and Discharge Planning, and Infection and Safety Control. She was an Activities Director at the Nursing Home and served as the first woman President of our local Lion's Club. Evelyn held diverse and challenging positions throughout her career and performed them well.

Between some of those roles, she had taken time off to be at home with the children and to enjoy life. Each time, she was able to resume a new position when she was ready to return to work. In about 1997, I recall when she resigned her position at the hospital as Infection Control and Safety Director and took three months off. After those months, she assumed a similar role in the nearby town of Asheboro. Before that time, she had always driven the car between the nearby communities comfortably and without concern. When she took the new position in Asheboro, she asked me to drive her to and from her job. Her request was very peculiar to me.

Most of our married life, Evelyn would come and go independently for shopping trips and errands. She began requesting more and more that I drive her. It was a significant change in her behavior. About that same time also, she stopped wanting to play Bridge with our neighbors whom we played with monthly. I found it odd that she would prepare the same meals three or four times in a row. All of her new behaviors were sending off subtle alarm bells in my head. There was nothing I could really put my mind around because the changes were so subtle. Besides, I am a man ... what can I say?

Not long after, she was terminated from her position in Asheboro. Evelyn explained to me that there was a conflict of personality with her boss. In looking back, I wonder if her ability to perform her job was already in question at that time.

Shortly thereafter, we elected to move as a family back to her home place in the North Carolina mountains. Evelyn and I agreed that she would work for about a year until I could restore her grandfather's home place. We would then run it as a bed and breakfast, which would create revenues that would sustain us. A year later, she still had not secured a job, and both of us were experiencing great stress. She did find a job as a floor nurse at a nursing home and was again terminated because she could not do the job quickly enough. She found another job at a local nursing home doing Infection Control and Safety and seemed to be doing reasonably well until she resigned to take an Industrial Nurse position. Once she had given her notice to the nursing home and gone to her new position, they decided they didn't want to hire her. She continued her job search and went to work at another nursing home. She worked for a day and a half, and they sent her home. None of these incidences had any effect on her. The terminations did not seem to faze Evelyn, and she never showed concern for her sub-par performance. She was content to be within her comfort zone at home.

Evelyn had always loathed watching television. She took pride in practicing personal hygiene, always being neat, and keeping a clean house. The situation eroded to her never bathing, cleaning the house, or cooking. She began to watch television four to eight hours a day. When she was not watching TV, she wanted to be right beside me all the time. It was driving me crazy. She was frustrated with me because she wanted to do things and could not. I was frustrated with her because I wanted to get things done. I could not be a caregiver and get the work done at the same time.

We were isolated, as Doris had been, with no one to help. For a period of time, I took Evelyn to Asheville, about 25 miles away, for Adult Daycare so I could have some relief.

I continued fulfilling my husband and caregiver roles to Evelyn, as well as being a caregiver to Carol. Then Evelyn became violent with my youngest daughter and me. Painfully, I recognized that something had to be done differently. It became obvious that it was time to put Evelyn in Assisted Living. We knew it would not be long before Carol would need 24-hour care as well, even though she was sharp cognitively.

It is here that Carol's and Evelyn's stories merge.

At Thanksgiving, I discussed with Carol that it was time to place Evelyn in Assisted Living and that I needed her help. This was a means to admit Carol into the care she needed also but would never acknowledge. I asked her if she would agree to accompany Evelyn and remain there with her for three months in the Assisted Living facility. If, after that time, Carol wanted to go back to Georgia, I would arrange it. The college left the apartment open for her to return if she desired. She agreed to the condition.

As well, I had to meet with Carol's General Practitioner to have him complete the FL2 admission forms for Assisted Living. I literally had to explain to him what Frontotemporal Dementia was and show him Carol's neurological and psychological evaluations. I got the feeling that he was not sure if I was on the up and up, but he completed the form as I requested. FTLD patients can disguise their condition, and in Carol's case, her intellect masked what was happening in her brain. Even her cousin thought nothing was wrong with Carol. Terri acted as my advocate in explaining to many of Carol's associates and friends that there truly was something significantly wrong with Carol. The key was that you had to speak with her for more than five minutes to be able to detect it. One of the coping mechanisms that FTD patients develop is to create little recordings in their minds that they can use over and over when needed. Those close to them can recognize the behavior because they repeat the information exactly the same every time.

Carol, Evelyn, and I went to her lawyer and drew up the legal documents needed for me to assist her. Those four documents were a will, a living will, financial power of attorney and health care power of attorney (see the Appendix for examples). All of this was completed in about an hour. The attorney needed to register the documents at the local county courthouse.

To place Evelyn and Carol together in Assisted Living, we had to reserve, or hold, a room in advance to assure that they could share a room. Of course, we had to bear these costs personally, as the insurance company does not pay benefits before a 90-day waiting period.

Initially, Carol agreed to accompany Evelyn, but chaos ensued. It was an emotional, roller coaster nightmare. For the next two months while I was solidifying the move for the two of them, Carol was vacillating daily. Yes, I will; no, I won't ... yes, I will; no, I won't. This, as so many caregivers know, is emotionally and psychologically catastrophic.

The time came for me to go to Georgia to lead Carol back to our home in the mountains. She was still driving a vehicle at that time and refused to come without her car. Additionally, I had to bring her computer, her baking equipment for bread, her personal library, sewing machine, and some of her wardrobe. She had developed strategies to allow her to do things, such as baking bread, operating her computer and sewing machine, as well as traveling from one location to another. She accomplished these by writing detailed, step by step notes. Sometimes the notes, pasted everywhere, were an inch thick. The morning we were to leave, she said, "No, I am not going." Desperate, I called on a Christian Psychologist friend who cajoled her by entreating her, "You need to do this for Evelyn." Finally, she got into the car and followed me to their childhood mountain home.

My youngest daughter and I prepared their new home quietly and with care to provide familiar decor that would make them feel at home. The next morning, Carol again refused to go, contrary to Evelyn who was compliant as a little child. To help me with Carol, I called on my personal friend and pastor for help.

I convinced Carol to accompany Evelyn, my daughter Anne, and me to a local restaurant to meet with my pastor and assistant pastor. Toward the end of the meal, my daughter and I left to finish the room preparation and admission process with the support personnel. Later that day, the pastor and assistant pastor brought Evelyn and Carol to the facility, and we took them to their new room and home. After explaining again why they were there, we quietly slipped away, leaving Evelyn and Carol to have prayer with the pastors. Unless you have lived through something like this, you cannot comprehend the pain.

Ironically, Carol has never asked to go home to Georgia and has stated that she could not imagine being there without her sister. She and Evelyn now share a room at the end of the hall (in the Assisted Living setting), just as they did when they were little girls.

There comes a time when the burden is too heavy and one must, for their own health and sanity's sake, allow others the privilege to care for their loved ones. Each caregiver has to personally make that decision when that time has arrived. You can believe me when I say that there will be people lined up telling you that you are wrong, whether you keep your loved one at home or choose to place them in assisted care. No matter what their opinion may be, they have not walked a mile in your shoes. As a caregiver, I know how difficult it is to come to this determination, and it has been my observation that many caregivers do not know when to let go. Guilt can reign supreme. For me, the decision to let go was when Evelyn became violent toward my youngest daughter and me.

Do not believe that you can place your loved one in assisted living or convalescent care on your own. You will need help. The decision may be difficult, but assistance will make the process easier. You will find beginning on page 114 of this book an article by Frances Coates, Administrator of the Marjorie McCune Memorial Facility, providing an excellent guide for caregivers on how and where to place your loved one in assisted care.

As it turned out, when Evelyn and I moved to the mountains of North Carolina, we jointly searched for employment opportunities for Evelyn. It happened to be that we visited the McCune Center as a prospective employer for her. Evelyn and I had both been active members of a local Lion's Club. The Lion's Club International, a phenomenal service organization, has thousands of local clubs throughout the world providing services for the blind and hearing impaired. The McCune Center is one of the few that is an assisted living facility, totally owned and operated by the local Lion's Club of Western North Carolina. What an absolute magical fit for Evelyn. To assist me in this transition, I met with Frances Coates and separately met with my pastor and assistant pastor to develop as easy a process as possible for admitting Evelyn and Carol.

It is essential that you, the caregiver, allow your loved one time to adjust to their new environment. It is vital that you NOT go back to see them for two or three weeks. Even though it is painful, it is essential for your emotional stability and for them to adapt to a new way of living. One key thing to understand when you have to take this defining step in releasing your loved one is that YOU deserve to move forward with your life.

After this period of adjustment, it is wise to refrain for a period of time, maybe even a year or two, from bringing them back to their previous dwelling for a visit. Stability is something they need, and instability is the enemy of their emotional balance. Even though there may be memory issues with your loved one, you are not doing them a favor by taking them back to long-established dwellings.

As of this writing, Evelyn and Carol have been in Assisted Living for four years. Last spring, we thought we would lose Carol to a complication of dehydration. Amazingly, she recovered and remains exceedingly cognizant and interactive. Remarkably, for the first time in my 40 years of knowing her, she actually appears happy. It is a delight to see her with this new persona.

As for Evelyn, my wife, even though they have the same disease and Evelyn is two years younger than Carol, Evelyn has deteriorated at an alarming rate. She no longer knows me or her children. When I visit her, she has a quizzical expression on her face, as if to say, "I know I should know who you are, but I just can't figure it out." I also believe that she is becoming aphasic (loss of ability to speak or understand language). When I ask her questions, she cannot process the answer but merely mimics my words. It is so very sad. This horrible Monster claims yet another dear one.

For Doris, Evelyn, and Carol, there is no hope. However, that is not the end of the story. ❖

Chapter 6
Anne's Story

We have now lived with and experienced three generations of family members wracked with this awful, nondiscriminating, debilitating disease (this Monster) that takes away the mind, memories, and motivations of some of the most kind, gentle, and intelligent people we have ever known. For those generations, when "going off" started at age 48 to 52, there was no going back. They would lose their dignity, their essence, and their family bonds to this menace. For us now, there is a fourth and possibly even a fifth generation. Until June 10, 2008, no one had expressed to us that there was any hope to stop or cure the advancing enemy that was this disease once the onset took place.

Let me tell you how blessed we are. Here is the chain of events: Doris, my mother-in-law, was taken to a physician in Siler City, instead of the more convenient process in Asheville, North Carolina. That initiated a sequence of contacts and events that today leads us to believe there is a reason to hope.

That event goes this way: from Siler City, Doris was sent to Duke University Memory Loss Clinic. Because she went to the Memory Loss Clinic, her brain tissue was donated to medical research, and no one will ever know how many will benefit from her contribution. As a result of our contact with the Memory Loss Clinic, Evelyn and Carol were enrolled in some scientific studies.

The awareness of this potential prompted me to protect myself by purchasing long term insurance, in case they actually did develop the disease. As an interested scientist, I persistently kept in contact with Dr. Gail V. W. Johnson, formerly of the University of Alabama, Birmingham, and presently at Rochester University in New York. She, in turn, referred me to Dr. John Hardy, then the Director of the National Institute of Health and Aging, who extended to us the opportunity to be tested in his research laboratory for the specific gene mutation that Doris had (FLTD-17 R406W Tauopathy). Subsequently, two of Evelyn's aunts—sisters of Doris—were tested to be positive. As a result of finding out this information, Dr. Hardy recommended that we speak with Dr. Brad Boevé at the Mayo Clinic in Rochester, Minnesota. Dr. Boevé offered us the opportunity to have my two daughters tested in his laboratory for the gene mutation.

To be able to receive the test results, the individuals must receive genetic counseling. As fortune would have it, Dr. Kirk Wilhelmsen had moved from California to the University of North Carolina at Chapel Hill. Dr. Wilhelmsen was a part of Dr. Mike Hutton's team that discovered the disease that haunts this family. Dr. Boevé recommended that Dr. Wilhelmsen be my daughters' genetic counselor. What a miraculous chain of events!

The results of the two tests were delivered to Dr. Wilhelmsen. He told my youngest daughter, Anne, that she had the gene and my oldest daughter, Donna, that she did not. Donna initially responded with great relief. After reveling in her good news, she noted the horror on Anne's face at not getting the same good news. Anne sat there stunned, as if hit by a cannon ball. Anne thought she was going to be spared because she did not look like Evelyn's family. We had prayed that both would be negative.

On June 3, 2008, Donna and Anne had their first consultation with Dr. Brad Boevé. Unlike previous generations with no hope, Dr. Boevé related to us that there is every reason to believe that interventions will be available before Anne comes to the usual age of the onset of this disease (48-52). A truly extraordinary chain of events! Truly, we are blessed. Added to our good fortune, Anne will be seen on an annual or bi-annual basis by Dr. Boevé at Rochester and Dr. Kaffure at UNC. Anne will have the phenomenal blessing of being treated by and exposed to the best science in the world for this disease.

We are hoping that when the time comes for Anne to have children that they will test negative and this monster's devastation will come to an end for our family.

We have shared with you four generations of the Monster that has been devouring our loved ones, and now we are ready to see science finally Slay the Monster. Amen! ❖

Chapter 7

Other Stories

*T*he following section is a compilation of stories from both caregivers and victims who have felt the attack of the Monster. We offer our heartfelt gratitude to each of them for taking their valuable time to share their often painful stories in an effort to give encouragement and let others reading this book know that they are not alone.

We have edited these stories for clarity, grammar, and punctuation but have tried to maintain the "voice" of those who are sharing.

Names and details have been changed in some of the stories to protect the families.

Jean's Story

My name is Jean Anderson, and I wanted to share my family's FTD story with you. I grew up in Cincinnati in a family of eight siblings in a very competitive, loud, and fun family.

In 1988, after graduating from college, I went to help my sister, Tina, in Long Island whose nanny needed to take time off. Tina and her husband had full-time careers and two children—a one-year-old son and six-year-old daughter. During my stay, I grew close to Tina and her family. For the first time as an adult, I got to know her because she was off to college and grad school by the time I was eleven. I was able to see various sides of Tina—the determined, creative, and caring business executive, the loving mother, and the terrific golfer. Eventually, their nanny returned, so I moved out and started by career in New York City.

Over the years, I stayed in close contact with Tina and her family, but I noticed a distance developing, as if she were surrounded by a wall and didn't want to let me in. When she was in her late 30s, I started telling my siblings that "something isn't right with Tina." They would ask me what I meant, and I would describe some behaviors I had noticed, such as purchasing too much food, buying things she didn't need, driving through stop signs (in a suburban town with lots of children), and not taking care of herself. They didn't agree with me, so I became more diligent and started keeping a list of strange behaviors. Eventually, she lost her job. Then her marriage started falling apart, and everything started to spin out of control. I got her involved with a therapist specializing in depression, whom she visited off and on (mostly off) for two years.

In January 1995, I received a disturbing call. Tina, who was living alone after her divorce, had been locked up against her will in a Psychiatric Hospital with a diagnosis of depression. Her neighbors had called the police several days after a snowstorm because they had not seen any signs of life, i.e., tire tracks, coming from her house. It was a terrible and frightening experience for Tina, but it was the catalyst for the family to come together and figure out what was going on. I took a hiatus from work for three months and was determined to find out what was wrong with her. After badgering the staff, we got Tina out of Bergen Pines in 17 days and received a bill from the hospital for $17,000.00 for locking her up against her will.

The therapist advised that Tina wasn't suffering from depression and recommended that we take her to a psychiatrist or neurologist. We went to a psychiatrist first—a big mistake. He diagnosed Tina with "simple schizophrenia" (a controversial diagnosis). After doing research, we decided to continue down the path of finding a world-class neurologist. We got her to the New York Hospital/Cornell Medical Center's Memory Disorders clinic. Thankfully, we were working with Dr. Alan Jacobs, who diagnosed her correctly with FTD. He explained that he couldn't guarantee that his diagnosis was 100% accurate without a brain biopsy, but he believed that the spect and pet scans, the changes in behaviors that I described (from my list that I'd been keeping), and the ruling out of all other possibilities gave him 95% confidence in his diagnosis. This occurred in 1996, after over a year's worth of testing, mainly because Tina wasn't cooperative in taking the various tests. It took approximately six years to get a diagnosis from when I started going public with "something isn't right with Tina." In retrospect, we were fortunate that she was diagnosed accurately because FTD was just beginning to be understood by the medical community. However, this experience of waiting years and going through multiple misdiagnoses seems to be the norm with FTD, which can be prevented through improved education and awareness for medical, social, and legal practitioners.

In the meantime, my sister, Karin, moved in with Tina, became primary caretaker, and got her life back in order.

Hearing that someone you love has been diagnosed with Frontotemporal lobe dementia (FTD) with "no treatment, no cure, and an average lifespan after diagnosis from 5 to 17 years" is worse than having an innocent person sentenced to prison for the rest of her life. But that is mild compared to what it's like to find out that the cause of FTD is an autosomal dominant gene, which occurs in approximately 10% of FTD cases.

After Tina's diagnosis, we talked about behavior similarities that Tina had with our mother (who died of breast cancer in 1991), and I was convinced that we needed to explore the possibility of a genetic cause, even though we knew of no other similar diseases in the family. My sister, Laura, and I spent time researching the top institutes who study FTD and convinced enough family members to participate in genetic research with UC-San Francisco in

2001 and the NIH in 2006. Neither institution found the gene through our blood samples. This gave us hope that our situation was not genetic. After all, only one out of nine siblings had the disease, and two top research institutes had not found anything genetic. The NIH also introduced us to a team at the Mayo Clinic led by Brad Boevé to help us figure out the genetics, but the family's interest level was low at the time given the lack of findings thus far.

Two things happened in the course of a year and a half to convince us to pursue the genetic research. In 2006, I received one of those "are you sitting down?" calls from Laura. She advised that she suspected another sibling, Patty, was displaying symptoms and shared her list of observed behavior changes over the past few years. Off we went to Omaha to work through another devastating marital and family situation. It was déjà vu all over again.

Then in 2007, our brother, Ted, received a letter from a distant relative asking, "Do you have any unusual diseases in your family?" We got in touch with our distant relatives, only to find out that FTD was prevalent on their side of the family, displaying an autosomal dominant gene pattern. It was like the launching of an atomic bomb!

This new information renewed the interest at the Mayo Clinic, so we made plans to participate in a double blind longitudinal study. Within a month of visiting the Mayo Clinic in 2008, they identified the genetic mutation. This was both a relief and a curse. Now we had information to go forth with clinical tests to find out if each individual has the gene or not. We were able to confirm the gene on our side of the family through the second sister we suspected of having FTD. Now the bomb had landed and exploded, and we are dealing with the nuclear fallout.

This difficult situation has given me the strength and determination to help advocate for the disease so we can find a cure before it takes another family member and devastates another family. I feel strongly that even though my family has been dealt a mighty blow, we can, will, and must do everything within our means to make a positive difference in the world because of this disease. We are participating in this longitudinal study in order to give researchers data to help find a cure. We are connecting with others who have the disease who want to educate public servants, such as the police officers who locked up my sister, due to his ignorance of dementia, and the psychiatrist who misdiagnosed her. We are volunteering for the Association for Frontotemporal Dementias (AFTD) to help advocate for the disease and help others who are seeking advice, information, and support. I am working with the Alzheimer's Association and the AFTD to understand how I can education legislators on this kind of dementia.

The most difficult part of this disease is the torture of slowly losing a loved one. Tina, who used to be a bright, capable, articulate leader is now nearly mute and needs someone to watch over her at all times. Her cognitive ability is on par with a one year old. When I look into her eyes, I still see Tina—the big sister who was my inspiration to keep my maiden name, to break the glass ceiling, and to balance my time across work, family, and community. I just wish I could have a conversation with the real Tina and talk about current events, her favorite memories of her children, or even just a joke. In some ways, I have already mourned her loss, but every time I see her, I hope that there will be a cure for her, as well as the 250,000 other "Tinas" out there suffering from FTD.

I am so grateful for the many medical and social workers who are helping families like ours deal with dementia—you are giving us hope. I would especially like to thank Dr. Boevé and his team at the Mayo Clinic and the AFTD. Without the support of these organizations and funding from the NIH, we would be much farther away from finding a cure. ❖

Caroline's Story

My name is Caroline Myers, and this is my story as a caregiver. It's hard to imagine that the roles of caregiving are so rapidly being reversed.

Two months before my mother's 70th birthday, it was determined that her frontal and temporal lobes were shrinking at an abnormally fast pace. The increased difficulty in accessing her language combined with a newfound access to her emotions were out of character for this formerly independent, articulate, and stoic mother of six, grandmother of 10, and wife of almost 50 years.

Soon before the diagnosis, she was the constant caregiver of everyone she loved. She will always be known as someone who would do, and did do, just about anything she could for her loved ones. We were all so accustomed to her commitment to going above and beyond to bring joy to others that the silent culprit of FTD was able to sneak up on us. Before we knew it, she was slipping away.

God has provided many blessings in this storm. I am honored and humbled to give back to my mother just a little of the caregiving she has bestowed upon me over the past 40 years of my life. There is nowhere I would rather be than piecing together a jigsaw puzzle with her. Although, the words between us are few, we enjoy a good hand bump each time we fit a piece together. I am hoping and praying that the Lord will help doctors and researchers piece together the puzzle pieces of this disease so that others in the future are spared the devastation that goes along with FTD. ❖

David's Story

*I*am David Griffith. The official start of my experience with the disease occurred with the pronouncement of the verified diagnosis that Sandra, my wife of 46 years, was between early-onset and mid-range Semantic Dementia.

For several years preceding this news, I had been supplying words for Sandra in her conversations. At the time, I thought it was just old age creeping in. It turns out that it was something much worse.

Since then, we all have been caught up in a constant search for answers and seeking desperately for someone to tell is it isn't so, or that something can be done to slow the continuing progression of this permanent fog bank that is blanking out the mind of our wife, mother, grandmother, and best friend. No answers, solutions, or real hope have been found as the fog progresses, closing her down.

We now cherish all of the events and moments that used to be taken for granted, the times we may never experience again the way we remember them in the past. Everything has a greater emotional content and intensity. We intend to love and treasure Sandra for all that she has been, is, and will be … even after the fog bank becomes permanent. ❖

Phyllis' Story: Is it Rockie, or Fred?

*J*ames "Rockie" McMakin was united in marriage to a woman certain she would never marry again after a failed first marriage with many major challenges, such as the first husband's critical motorcycle accident with brain injury, drugaddiction, alcoholism, and "going off." The best thing she had from that 11-year marriage was a beautiful daughter.

At first date, reticent woman knew that this man was her very life to be. After two months, they exchanged vows after personally vowing never to be unfaithful and never to divorce, no matter what. The beautiful little daughter immediately held out her arms to new "Daddy" Rockie on January 1978. Daddy Rockie loved being her father and said he would like to have a son. We immediately conceived, and I told Daddy Rockie I guaranteed a BIG BOY! He was pulled into the world on October 6, 1978, weighing 8 pounds 13 ounces, with a 14 ¾-inch head and 15-inch shoulders. Right away, he proceeded to tear down the temperature probe in the incubator, and his 23-inch length filled the crib.

Our life was made up of dance lessons, soccer, t-ball, softball, drill team, football, band, honor choir, Lt. Governor of Key Club, and up through Boy Scouts to Life Award. What busy days we had, but time was always available to be together at breakfast and dinner as a family. And, oh, the glorious weekends and vacations. Our favorite times were visiting Hot Springs National Park, a complete tour of all the State Parks of Oklahoma, Roaring River Missouri, a complete circle of all regions of Texas, a plane trip to San Marcos, and the glass bottom boats. What fun we had, with Rockie doing most of the driving and me navigating.

Working for the State gave us little take-home pay after deductions for Social Security, State Retirement, and health and life insurance. But, boy, did we get nice holidays with our families. I was District Director for the Texas Public Employees Association, so when the Texas Legislature said they had no money for pay raises, we said give us another holiday, pay our health insurance premiums, and get us prescription drug coverage. They did! This proved to be so valuable to us, especially Rockie and me.

Rockie was a Social Services Worker II, and I was a Social Services

Supervisor II when he got his first "Meets Requirements" annual review. He had been "Outstanding" his entire career since 1974. He was devastated and puzzled.

This formerly outstanding employee was not able to learn the new computer system, and the supervisor had given him a list of cases that he did not complete with his regular outstanding workmanship. Then I noticed he was stopping at green traffic lights and once took off in the middle of a red light … me screaming for him to STOP!

Other things started to happen, severe depression (with some vague reference to killing himself) and not being able to find his way back to the office from home visits. He became flat emotionally, and it was hard for the children or me to get a response from him. Then we suspected what we had dreaded for many years, the same "whatever it was" that his two uncles, one aunt, and his father suffered. The doctors just said it was not Alzheimer's, but it was something that caused them to retire early, be depressed, and … eventually lose their minds.

Now, the not-so-fun part of our "forever life" began. There were trips to personal Doctor Stock to check out what could be wrong. All body parts checked out fine, except low, low iron, so B-12 shots began … no intrinsic factor. That could be causing some of the memory problems. Then we had a referral to a local neurologist, Dr. Harrison. Rockie came back, sat across my desk from me, and said, "The one appointment you missed with me is when they found something, and the doctor wants you to call him immediately."

I called, and what the doctor told me did not really sink in. I called him back the next day and listened through tears and sobs coming from deep within as he stated that Rockie was to retire immediately, and that he was in danger of driving off, thinking he could find his way home by walking, and we would never see him again. Dr. Harrison said there were no brain waves in a part of his brain and that he would have to go to Southwestern Medical School in Dallas or Baylor Neurology in Houston. He referred us to Baylor Neurology, and Rockie was scheduled to see Dr. Eugene Lai in early September.

Rockie immediately took medical leave (the valuable thing I told you about earlier) and was on full pay until the medical leave ran out, which was about 30 days. In the meantime, we traveled to Houston for a long week of medical tests.

On the weekend before the tests began, Rockie and I made plans for the rest of our lives. We cried a lot for the first time, and I told him I would never put him in a nursing home unless absolutely necessary, that I would tie him to a tree or use a dog zapper if he wandered off (kidding of course). We decided we would live as normal a life as possible. Remember, Rockie and I were both Social Workers, so we made our own Case Management and determined not to let this "Stuff" ruin our lives. I would take over all the financial functions, and we would go to an attorney and have powers of attorney drawn up and a new will.

The tests began. They checked everything again. Heart, lungs, blood for all kinds of known genetic diseases, AIDS, a spinal tap, and finally, a sleep study and EEG. First, 24 hours and then about 16 more hours of having electrical patches all over Rockie's head, chest, and legs. Dr. Lai scheduled us to come back in two weeks.

Rockie was plunging fast into a black pit. Ryan, Donetta, and I had to pull him back. He sometimes went into rages over frustration with himself for what he could not do. I told Ryan if he wanted to learn about cars and engines and things, he had better start immediately to have his father teach him before he forgot.

My father cried with me when I told him the outcome of the tests, and my Mother, in her usual way, at first denied anything being wrong, but then confessed that she had seen changes.

Everyone was curious about the illness. Most friends said they did not think it was true. He seemed normal to them. They did not know how we prepared Rockie for every event, telling him who would be there, what we would be doing, practicing with him what to say, and picking out his attire. He continued to lead music at church but would get very short and angry when he messed up, storming out and sometimes throwing his book down. He became more and more compulsive in his behavior and more outspoken. We sometimes cringed when he acted inappropriately or said the wrong thing. When he had an excessively bad day, my son and I started calling him "Fred," which has become our code word for him not acting right or to call his attention to his bad behavior.

I continued to work, as we were on half our previous income with no Social Security or State Disability yet. When I call home to check on him, he would have forgotten to eat anything. I would find that he could not account for his time. So the doctor suggested we keep him on a schedule. I would call around lunch time and remind him where I put his food in the refrigerator. He just was no longer the Rockie I had married; most of the time he was Fred.

He fully trusted me and his children. Had he not done so, I think our life would have been a big loss. We continued to love each other, and I hid nothing from Rockie. We were always up front about his dementia, remembering going to the funerals for his uncle, age 85, who had no communication the last five years of his life in the nursing home, and his aunt who lived to 82 and had spent the last twelve years of her life not knowing where she was or her own children. She had started the symptoms of the disease about age 62, his uncle at age 56, and his dad at age 55. Only one sibling of his dad's was unaffected. The uncle who died in his fifties in a nursing home had complained for several years that there was something wrong. He had dementia and died in a nursing home with cancer. Rockie's dad had tremors in his hand, depression, tiredness, was not able to drive, head bobbing yes, and flat emotional effect. He had to retire at 56 because he could not do his job, physically or mentally. He died from complications of radiation for cancer at age 66.

Rockie keeps a journal, and marks off his day. He putters around in his shop and is working on his Dodge pickup, having put in a more powerful motor. He works on lawnmowers for neighbors. He may work all day, but only charges for parts he uses.

His hoarding of old parts has recently become a problem; our son kept saying that his dad was keeping trash. At first, I thought he meant old trash parts. Well, he was doing that, too, but was literally saving trash—old waded up papers, old paper boxes, old empty paint cans. I hired Joe to clean for three solid days in Rockie's shop; the first night Joe stopped at 5:15 p.m., and by 7:00 p.m., Rockie had it nearly all back in the shop. We are still working on the hoarding issue. I have made him watch the hoarding show on TV.

Since 1994, we have made two to three trips a year to Dr. Lai in Houston. He says Rockie is one of his successful patients, of which there are few. As of this writing, we have been to Houston twice in the last two months and have an appointment on August 24 for PET Scan, a sleep study, and an EEG.

Our son and daughter have both finished their college degrees and are successful, responsible grownups who love their Daddy Rockie very much.

Our son has a wife and stepson. They are thinking of having another child, but want to know if he is a carrier of a genetic mutation. I could have had him tested for free by Texas Tech when he was in high school, but I was afraid it would influence his future life too much.

Our daughter and her husband have a beautiful five-month-old daughter, Olivia, who has put a new passion in her Grandpa Rockie's life. When it comes to me, Rockie still treats me as the queen of his life, and we have a deeper love than ever. I never see Fred when I look in his eyes. And his children don't see Fred either, only the strong love of a Daddy and a Grandpa.

Phyllis S. McMakin, soon to be married 33 years to my Rock! Rockie. ❖

Marlene's Story

"A sister is a gift to the heart, a friend to the spirit,
a golden thread to the meaning of life."
—Isadora James

My sister, Kathleen, is indeed a gift to me, but she is also a gift to all who know and love her. The thought of watching my sister and friend go away from me so quickly, before my very eyes, is a difficult task. It is something that this disease does; it strips our loved one of their uniqueness as a person, that person that we love so dearly. The only way to cope with the hurt, for me, is to get involved with finding ways to cure this dreadful disease and give support to those who are facing this reality.

Kathleen has the disease called "Frontotemporal Dementia," sometimes referenced as PICK's disease. As the name implies, it affects the frontal and temporal lobes of the brain. The first signs of the disease are so gradual that it is extremely hard to determine what is going on with your loved one. It is not only the family members who have questions, the doctors also have a hard time identifying the disease. The primary diagnosis from visiting the doctor is that the patient is depressed, and they prescribe an anti-depressant medicine. When this does not help, the long, drawn out doctor visits start, and, with Kathleen, she would always come back from the visits with a "clean bill of health." But as family members, we knew differently.

The first sign of the disease was an extreme personality change, which included behavior, ability to reason, ability to make decisions, ability to handle anything dealing with math, no longer interested in personal appearance, and more. These were the primary issues that were affecting Kathleen, but there was not one doctor who could identify the problem! It became an almost five-year journey from one doctor to another.

Finally, in September 2008, a neurologist recognized what "could be" FTD-PPA and started Kathleen on some meds that would help her anxiety. The family was heartbroken when we started understanding the outcome of this diagnosis. There is no cure for this disease, and after the diagnosis, the usual lifespan is five to ten years.

We were able to get Kathleen into the National Institute of Health in Maryland in February 2009, at which time the diagnosis was confirmed. After a week and a half of testing, Dr. Wassermann reviewed the findings with us for about 30 minutes. He recommended getting respite care to come into the home at least three to four times per week for the well being of Kathleen's husband, Leo, and Kathleen. The doctor also told us that Kathleen was not allowed to ever drive a vehicle again. Kathleen made no response to this news. She had a blank look on her face the whole time he was talking, looking off into space, chewing her gum. She had several of the symptoms of all of the FTD dementias, not only the dementia that the local physician named (PPA – Progressive Primary Aphasia).

As we read and learned more about this disease, I wanted to share it with the Human Resource Directors and Associates at our Church for one reason: Kathleen is not only my sister but, in my humble opinion, one of the best Human Resource Directors in our Church! She took the Carolina Conference from "scratch" and built a model example of how to keep the vital records in the order needed for easy access as well as security. Kathleen also held the title of Associate Secretariat. She was admired by the Carolina Conference Officers for her ability to "just handle the situation" and keep the Officers up to date on needed information without having to worry them with details. It became very difficult to accept when the work was not excellent, when the attitude was not always excellent, when the numbers were not calculated correctly. Kathleen had been admired by our Legal Counsel for her abilities to deal with extremely sensitive issues with the expertise of the "best"!

It is now March 2010 at the time of this writing. The year of 2008 will always be remembered by my family. It was the year of tragedy. In February 2008 my mother-in-law passed away at the age of 85. She lived a full life, but it is never easy to say good-bye for now. In April 2008 my brother died from pancreatic cancer that was not diagnosed until February 2008! Next, in September 2008, Kathleen was diagnosed with FTD. In October 2008, Kathleen's husband, Leo, was laid off from his full-time job! To say the year was unrivaled would only be the tip of the iceberg! The year of 2009 seemed to be filled with recovery from the four major blows and almost a blur in recalling particular instances.

In the aftermath of finding out Kathleen's diagnosis, my sister-in-law, Faye (wife of the brother that died from cancer in April 2008) and I, visited the Cary, North Carolina, FTD Support Group in November 2008. The group was small, probably seven to eight people plus Faye and myself, but it does not take volume in numbers to be heard! It was so therapeutic to be able to talk with people who were "nodding their heads in understanding"! For us it was refreshing to be able to openly voice our frustration about the amount of time it took to find a doctor with the correct diagnosis, and so many other issues. It was so obvious to me that we "needed" to have a support group in Charlotte!

I talked with the facilitator, Charlene, that evening before leaving. She encouraged me to consider being the facilitator for Charlotte. My immediate and very sincere answer was, "No, we have to have someone like yourself who knows the disease." Charlene called the National FTD headquarters, and I later received a call from Sharon Denny, Programs Director for AFTD – Association of Frontotemporal Dementia. After much discussion, Sharon convinced me to accept this challenge, which I wholeheartedly embraced.

Do you know how to mend a broken heart? The reason I ask the question is simple. My heart was broken. I could not find a way to cope with the terrible loss of my best friend, my sister, my co-worker, my lunch partner. I am a Christian that had poured out my heart and soul to the Lord to intervene and for the "peace of mind" to accept His Will. I very often found myself in a heap of tears and prayed that I could overcome my grief to be useful to others with similar suffering. So, do you know the answer? It is simple … take your broken heart and start "reaching out to others and help them find peace"! Yes, it is that simple, and it works in ways that only the Lord will know. But, my dear friends, it works!

January 2009, on the second Sunday of the month, the first Charlotte FTD Support Group met. We have not missed one month since that time. My broken heart is mending! Suffice it to say, it will always have an empty spot from my loss of Kathleen, but my heart is healing!

Kathleen, the professional, well-spoken, empathetic, intelligent person that we knew and loved so dearly, is no longer the same person. She needs 24/7 care now. She has a blank, expressionless look. She no longer talks, although she still has the ability. She paces the floor all day long. Kathleen will not sit down to eat but will grab a bit of food and continue to pace the floor. She can assist with minor duties, such as taking the dishes to and from the table. Other than minor tasks, Kathleen does nothing! She stopped reading about three years ago. Even the flicking of the television channels with the remote has stopped. She has to be helped with her daily routine of bathing and getting dressed. Kathleen will be 62 in April 2010. So young! She had so many dreams to accomplish, and now her sweet and dedicated husband, Leo, is doing all he can to simply make her comfortable.

What do we expect? As a family, we have learned that expectations are limited. By the grace of God, we have learned to cherish each moment, do only things that will give Kathleen a peaceful day, and when we lay to rest each night, know that God Almighty only has the answers. In the meantime, we press on, loving her and one another. We aspire to make a difference in others' lives by supporting them in their grief and pain until this horrible disease will be a thing of the past. ❖

Susan's Story

Losing my mind, losing my personality, losing me.
—Susan L. Grant

My greatly adored grandfather said to tell people what you think of them while they are alive. I enjoy those people who are so surprised by my telling them about some of their traits that I have valued the most in our friendships. We live this fragile life trying to be the best we can be. It's not easy looking someone in the eye and saying, "You're the most honest and ethical person I know." Their reactions tell me they aren't used to hearing good things.

What matters most in my life right now is that people are thanked and know how they have touched me. My diagnosis is a deteriorating, terminal brain disease, FTD with parkinsonian symptoms. Being newly diagnosed, people have started telling me what they think of me, and it has helped. Others have denied that I am sick and don't even want to discuss it. That makes me angry; I feel like I am losing my mind, losing my personality, and losing me.

If I only had seeping blood from my left temporal lobe … I would be so grateful. It would seem more real! We could judge it a good or bad day by how much was flowing. I have good days that come and go. There isn't really any activity that helps bring the blessed few good ones. It is often as though the sun just came out from behind the clouds. The sky is bright blue, and birds sing their hearts out. I raise my hands toward the sky in a thankful, cheerful expectation for the day. My good, clear days are lessening, and they may last only a few hours.

Bad days are often following days that I overdid, or was upset. The sun is not out. I don't even think about how much beauty there was on the good day. I don't think about much but try to save my energy. It would be nice to take a nap to just relax. Relaxation is not a sensation that comes very often. I might not be crawling out of my skin, but the relentless buzzing is there. Even most mornings when I wake up aching, I try hard to have a "can do" attitude. Sometimes it works.

On really good days, I question if this disease is real. If I get three-four good days in a row, I drift back to fantasize that perhaps I will be okay. The next day is excruciating to get through because reality always returns. Tears flow from that endless well. I believe this is one of the hardest parts about a degenerative disease. Grieving goes on and on. You deal with one loss, and the next one rears it ugly head. I am losing capabilities of my brain quickly. Somehow the disease becomes more real each time.

Losing things, other than the keys ... Everyone talks about senior moments. Listen to your friends with bad memories. So as you discuss symptoms, they will chime in with all kinds of examples, trying to tell you that you are not alone, that they know what it is like. It's more difficult than that, and I wish they understood. I can feel my mind fading away. Then what will be left? If you thought you were just going to be mute, sit, and review all the fun experiences in life, that might be okay to endure for a few years. But my anxiety and confusion seem to dampen that spirit.

Slowly this disease steals your abilities, one by one. Thinking used to be one of my favorite things. I got paid, as a financial advisor, to think, to see the big picture with clients, to analyze numbers and then add a huge dose of common sense, which I did very well. Out would come topics for them to consider and alternatives to their situation from which they could choose. Often they would just want me to give them the answer. I had the confidence and knowledge to do that for large, important decisions in others' lives. To my devastation, I had to tell a friend the other day that she could not trust me in my advice about financial matters anymore. My heart ended up in my throat.

Oh, to think fast again and, most importantly, to multi-task. Verbal sparring and getting my point of view across has always been great fun, and I took it as an art form—the art of persuasion. It was one of my favorite pastimes with associates as we discussed crucial issues and, in turn, sharpened our skills. Perhaps now I need a "handicap" assigned to still participate. I don't think as fast as I used to, I have slowed on many things. Now, I am lucky to get the next word out. My face turns red, all the way down to my toes, when I cannot find a word or finish a thought. I am mixing their usage, turning them around as though the Scrabble board was multi-dimensional in my mind.

And the communication piece, the reaction to a possibility of becoming mute … People proudly come up with a solution of sign language or pointing to pictures … great; what a life, all that I have strived for over my lifetime will be different … it will be "crude." What a change! I have tried to develop skills to learn technical processes, people skills—studying them to know what they are thinking and needing, to be a good person, to have my word count 100%, what I have wanted the most in all the competitive worlds I have achieved—always getting better and doing my personal best. The shades of gray in my clients' lives have made the difference. Part of the time I was over achieving because of guilt, partly from the challenging of others, by far the most came from my own expectation that I could do almost anything I wanted as long as I put in the time and effort. I was such an overachiever for my own sake.

I get to the point of overloaded and can't think, make a choice, or even get a sound out. When I am driven too fast around town, I can become very disoriented and anxious. Sometimes my brain gets clogged and will not process for several seconds, even though it seems like minutes. It then has to take the question in and do something with it, which seldom comes out right at that point. It is easier to just say no thank you to whatever might have been offered than to think about the answer.

Many people have their own agenda for me. They want me to continue with grace and dignity, then leave with the same way! You've got to give it all you've got. Fight it to the end. You can beat this one. Let's not give you any other idea by what we say. We increase your depression if we talk about it. What do we say next if we ask how you are doing and it is not good? Their motivation is all wrapped in emotions, of course. But …

Losing so many things completely is like dying one piece at a time. Eventually, I will be like a zombie. I think about that a lot. Do I exist if there is no past that I can remember? And if I have no thoughts about what I will be doing tomorrow? So if I live five to ten more years, what will they be like? So far it is hell feeling so extremely fatigued. The aching is no fun. Am I still living as a zombie, or do I cease to exist sometime before that, leaving only a body behind. It seems as though you would like to just fade away. If you can't think, is that existing? If I can think and communicate for only two more years, and then live another eight, is that a good thing?

Hurry, the Lights are Going Out, fading away, everything is changing. What if there isn't enough time to …

To think, remember, reason, communicate, do things quickly, concentrate, relay feelings and continue adding to society, these are things I will miss the most. These are part of the things that make me different from everyone else. They define my personality and me. I am losing me.

I can be doing nothing, and a wave of anxiety comes over me. Why? I was not thinking of anything particularly sad, challenging, or depressing. I could tell it was the disease … brain chemistry … which is the catch, you can't will it to leave. People tell me to "just relax, listen to soft music, take a hot shower, get a grip." Some may be thinking, "You must be taking pity on yourself or thinking about your dying. What a wimp." With our society, this makes a comment on your constitution. I challenge that thinking. Surely, if I could get the disease to release its grip, I would give anything!

There is oftentimes much anxiety, frustration, and fear. Imagine these feelings, only stronger and intensified many times. It feels like a bolt of extreme energy in your body vibrating in each muscle incessantly. My limbs are frozen and tingling. I experience a fear that is like no other. It doesn't make sense, and there doesn't seem a way to back out of it. It is pure terror. I can barely catch my breath, my stomach is tied in knots, and I feel as though I want to crawl out of my skin. The loss of the feeling of control is so strong that my mind wanders in many different avenues. This is certainly not what I describe as a good day. The tingling through my body is very aggravating. Even the tips of my fingers tingle. At this point, it is nice to have people understand that it is physiological or organic, not something psychological. I did not produce it. My disease was not caused by overworking, burnout, or any thing I have done. I say it's nothing to get mad at God about; it's just biology.

Modern miracles of science have given me medications that help a lot. The reason I emphasize anxiety with dementia is that my mother had it several years ago, and I did not know what it was to get her help. I would walk in her nursing home and see people with a "wild look" in their eyes or pacing down the halls. I felt for these people suffering when medication could calm them and help them feel better.

Guilt, apathy, flat-lining, where did my highly motivated self go? What about the caring, extremely passionate feelings? One of the things I feel most guilty about is that I just don't feel like doing much. One of the functions of the frontal lobe is motivation. It seems now, one of my greatest loses. My enthusiasm is lessening, I call it "flat-lining." My caregiver has enough to deal with, let alone me not being upbeat. Lucky for me she has more energy bottled for me to use. I feel guilty she had to quit her job. I know her emotions, and she is hurting, which I feel bad about. She didn't sign up for this disease, nor did I. So much coordination. At the same time, I am so grateful to her. I try to share often what I am feeling, which seems helpful.

I have heard people talking about flat-lining, as though they were doing so on purpose, not responding to the caregiver's needs. That is so turned around. I feel myself not taking action, not caring, in a zombie state. I want to get out of it, but it just doesn't come. I absolutely know that I am not my old self but dearly wish I could have that old personality back! ❖

THE 10 PROGRESSIVE DEMENTIAS

1. **Late-onset Alzheimer's Disease**

2. **Early-onset Alzheimer's Disease**

3. **Dementia with Lewy Bodies**

Frontotemporal Lobar Dementia (FTLD):

   4. FTLD Behavioral variant

   5. FTLD Corticobasal degeneration

   6. FTLD with Motor Neuron disease

   7. FTLD Pick's disease

   8. FTLD Progressive Aphasia

   9. FTLD Semantic Dementia

   10. FTLD Progressive Supranuclear Palsy

❖ ❖ ❖

Distribution of the Progressive Dementias

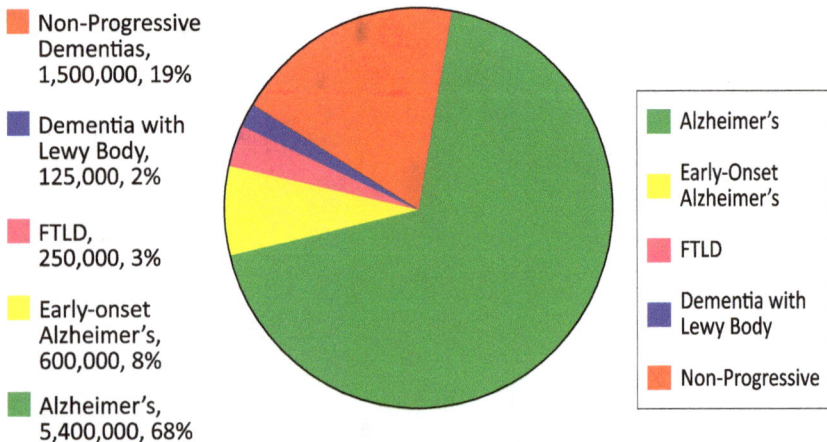

Non-Progressive Dementias, 1,500,000, 19%

Dementia with Lewy Body, 125,000, 2%

FTLD, 250,000, 3%

Early-onset Alzheimer's, 600,000, 8%

Alzheimer's, 5,400,000, 68%

Alzheimer's

Early-Onset Alzheimer's

FTLD

Dementia with Lewy Body

Non-Progressive

Chapter 8

Overview of the Dementias

*W*hat is known about dementias is always changing. New information that is being gathered by the scientific community is a major part of the changing names of diseases, how the diseases are presented, and how diseases are placed into groupings. The following is a discussion by the author concerning a portion of the "ftd-picks.org" website. Our intent is to help the reader understand this scientifically difficult text.

In 2009, **The Association for Frontotemporal Dementias** revised their website [www.ftd-picks.org]. Two changes were made to the original website as noted below.

1. **Lewy Body Dementia** was removed from being a part of Frontotemporal Lobar Degeneration (FTLD). It was felt by physicians and the scientific consulting group for AFTD, that Lewy Body Dementia was not a part of this dementia disease group. We will follow their lead and place Lewy Body Dementia as a separate disease in the **Progressive Dementias** along with Alzheimer's Diseases and the FLTD group of diseases.

2. In the previous website model, there was a designated group labeled **FTLD-17**. Two different types of diseases were noted from chromosome 17. They were designated as **FTLD-17 tau** and **FTLD-17 progranulin**. Both diseases are caused by different gene errors on chromosome 17. These two disease groups are now designated as **FTLD-Microtubular Associated Tau Protein (MAPT)** and **FTLD-Progranulin (PGRN)**. Each of these is discussed in the "genetic" portion of the revised website as detailed below.

Because of their unique nature of being inheritable, FTLD-MAPT are the tauopathies, and FTLD-PGRN are the Progranulin TDP-43 mutations. They are NOT shown as individual FTLD diseases. If you are interested in more details, go to the FTD-Pick.org website and read the "Genetics" section.

In the Science section of this text, you will note that there is a discussion about the 453 gene mutations and the faulty proteins associated with the dementias. Two of those sections are #4) the MAPT tauopathies (66 gene mutation types), and #5) is the PGRN TDP-43 (TARDBP) gene mutations (123 gene mutation types).

Progressive Dementias, diseases of neurons

*P*rogressive dementias are caused by diseased neurons. They have a time of onset, and after the onset, they become worse until the patient expires. Progressive dementias have a cause that may be either partially known or not fully understood. Three types of progressive dementias are:

- **Alzheimer's Disease (AD)**
- **Frontotemporal Lobar Dementia (FTLD)**
- **Dementia with Lewy Body (DLB)**

I. **Alzheimer's disease**, the first type of progressive dementia, is sub-divided into two different types: **early-onset** and **late-onset** Alzheimer's disease. Both forms have similar symptoms, even though the course of the disease may be somewhat different. Three differences between early-onset and late-onset Alzheimer's are the age of onset, the types of genes associated with the disease, and the longevity of the disease.

II. **Frontotemporal Lobar (Dementia) Degeneration (FTLD)** is the second type of progressive dementia. The FTLD group includes seven (7) different clinical subtypes of the disease that initially affects the frontal and temporal areas of the brain and inevitably progresses until the patient dies. These subtypes of FTLD are as follows:

1. **Behavioral variant (bv)** characterized by changes in personality, or exaggerations of one's personality.

2. **Corticobasal degeneration (CBD)**. Even though muscle strength remains normal, it is a movement disorder with muscle rigidity and tremors. Cognition is often affected.

3. **FTLD with Motor Neuron Disease (MND)**. This is also known as FTLD - Amyotrophic Lateral Sclerosis (ALS) or Lou Gehrig's disease. Muscle rigidity, behavior, language, and muscle control and muscle strength are affected with rigidity.

4. **FTLD Pick's disease.** This was the first FTLD disease recognized. Social, language, and personality are affected, making it difficult to distinguish from FTLD Behavioral variant, Aphasia, and Parkinson's. Findings of "Pick Bodies" at autopsy often confirms the diagnosis.

5. **FTLD Progressive Aphasia** (also known as Progressive Nonfluent Aphasia (PNFA). Patients with Progressive Aphasia have deterioration in their ability to speak because of a loss of the knowledge of grammatical organization and the ability to make sounds of language.

6. **FTLD Semantic Dementia (SD)** is a disorder of language such that there is loss of understanding words or objects. Other cognitive faculties may remain intact. These individuals can speak but cannot remember the word and often cannot remember the meaning of words.

7. **FTLD Progressive Supranuclear Palsy (PSP)** at its core is a visual disorder with a progressive inability to coordinate eye movements. This disease is also related to Parkinson's. PSP is the only FTLD that is not progressive to death. Because of the visual difficulties, gait and balance are significantly affected.

III. **Dementia with Lewy Bodies (DLB)** is a third type of progressive dementia. It is a type of dementia closely allied with both Alzheimer's and Parkinson's diseases. It is characterized anatomically by the presence of Lewy Bodies, clumps of alpha-synuclein and ubiquitin protein in neurons. Lewy Body Dementia victims typically have hallucinations and depression.

Non-Progressive Dementias, death of neurons

These cases of dementia are **not diseases of neurons**, but **death of neurons** due to either mechanical injury or some physiological process. This group of dementias, even though incapacitating, does not generally progress to death.

Accidents can cause brain injures that mimic dementia. This group includes brain damage caused by trauma—accidents or wounds that are mechanically induced.

Physiologically induced dementias include **Vascular Dementia**. Even though strokes are referred to as Cerebral Vascular Accidents (CVA), we chose to put vascular dementia into this physiological group. Vascular dementias are also called multi-infarct disease (strokes).

Another consideration for physiologically induced dementia may be **vascular constriction**, as in diabetes. Other causes of physiological dementia of the vascular nature may be a deprivation of blood supply by aneurisms or tumors, as well as blood clots and cholesterol plagues. The author is unable to decide where to put Transic Ischemic Attacks (TIAs). ❖

Chapter 9

The Progressive Dementias

Diseased neurons

- **Early- and Late-onset Alzheimer's Diseases (AD)**
  - **Frontotemporal Lobar Dementias (FTLD)**
    - **Dementia with Lewy Body (DLB)**

I. Alzheimer's Disease (AD)

Early-onset Alzheimer's Disease (EAD)

Cases of dementia diagnosed with **familial** AD before the age of 65 are known as Early-onset Alzheimer's Disease. It is an uncommon form of Alzheimer's accounting for only 0.1-10% of all Alzheimer's sufferers. Half of the early onset Alzheimer's cases are Familial Alzheimer's disease (FAD) cases, meaning there is a genetic predisposition to get the disease. Familial early-onset Alzheimer's can be diagnosed as early as 16 years of age. These early onset cases share the same traits as do the late-onset form of Alzheimer's. The remaining half of those diagnosed with early-onset Alzheimer's disease are non-familial, "sporadic" early-onset Alzheimer's (SAD). A sporadic case means that the individual does not have a family history of dementia and no genetic cause is suspected. Non-familial "sporadic" early-onset Alzheimer's can develop in people who are in their 30s or 40s, but it is extremely rare. The majority of early-onset patients are in their 50s or early 60s. Early-onset Alzheimer's is caused by a set of Autosomal Dominant genes. The three errant gene mutations result in the body manufacturing abnormal Presenilin 1 and 2 and Amyloid Precursor Proteins. The genes in early-onset Alzheimer's appear to be a different set of genes than those associated with late-onset Alzheimer's.

Late-onset Alzheimer's disease (LAD)

Late-onset Alzheimer's disease (LAD) is the most common form of dementia. Between 75-85% of all dementias are late-onset Alzheimer's. **This progressive, degenerative disease afflicting patients over 65 is incurable and terminal.** In 1906, Alois Alzheimer, a German psychiatric and neuro-pathologist was the first to recognize this malady as a unique disease. Thus, it bears his name. It is estimated that there are approximately 6 million individuals afflicted with this disease in the United States and greater than 35 million worldwide. Predictions are that these numbers will reach over 107 million in the U.S. by 2050 and that the care of these patients will potentially bankrupt our health care system.

The defining characteristics of an individual with Alzheimer's is initially short-term memory loss. Often, caregivers are alerted by this symptom and carry their loved one to a physician. Most often, the individual realizes that there is something going wrong as well. A physician will use various methods to confirm a diagnosis of Alzheimer's. This evaluation may include behavioral assessments, cognition examinations, and possibly brain scans. As the disease progresses, language skills and long-term memory decline. Behaviorally, the AD patient may become more irritable, aggressive, and unpredictable. As their abilities deteriorate, they become more withdrawn and eventually are unable to perform even normal activities of daily living (ADL), such as brushing teeth, hygiene, preparing a meal, or doing housecleaning. In the final stages, the individual must be cared for 24/7 and may progress to a catatonic state before death takes them. The average life expectancy after diagnosis is approximately seven years.

The consensus of the scientific community is that the combination of genetics and environmental factors cause this dementia. Genetically, abnormal proteins (**amyloid plaques**) accumulate between the glial structure between the neurons, and tangled bundles of fibrils (**neurofibrillary tangles**) accumulate within the neurons. **These two factors contribute to the cause of Alzheimer's disease (AD).** Scientists also believe that the genes of apolipo-protein (APOE) located on chromosome 19 contributes to an increased risk

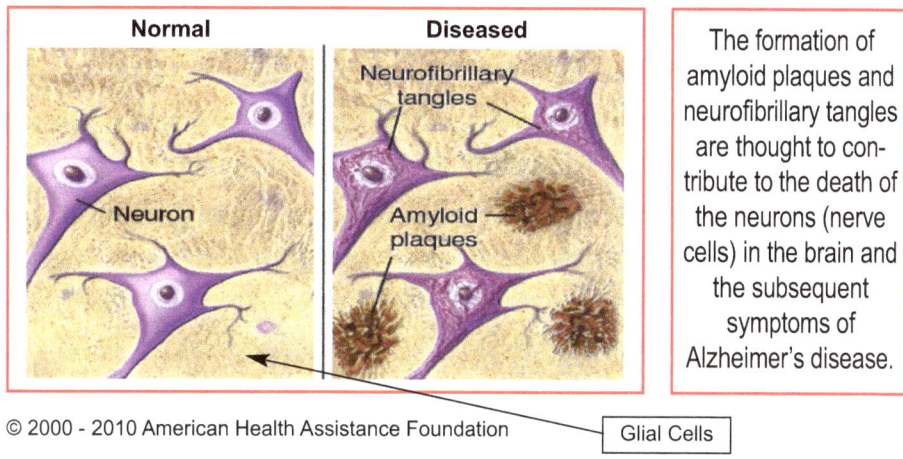

Normal	Diseased

The formation of amyloid plaques and neurofibrillary tangles are thought to contribute to the death of the neurons (nerve cells) in the brain and the subsequent symptoms of Alzheimer's disease.

Glial Cells

of developing late-stage Alzheimer's. The APOE has three common forms or alleles APOE ε2, APOE ε3 and APOE ε4. If an individual has two copies of the APOE allele ε4, there is a 15 times greater risk of developing Alzheimer's, and their symptoms accelerate compared to other Alzheimer's patients. It is conceivable that scientists will discover even more abnormal genes and proteins that contribute to developing Alzheimer's as they continue their search for a cure.

There are presently no drugs that *significantly* alter the course of the disease or management of the care of the individual. The drugs that are available are commonly known to only temporarily provide some improved cognition. But, after a period of time, the dementia progresses even with the medications.

Amyloid Plaques

One of the hallmarks of Alzheimer's disease is the accumulation of **amyloid plaques** among the **glial cells** in the brain. Glial cells provide the framework of the brain, while it is the neurons that enable the brain to work. "Amyloid" is a general term for protein fragments that the body produces normally. **Beta amyloid** is a protein fragment snipped from **amyloid precursor protein (APP)**. In a healthy brain, these protein fragments are broken down and eliminated by the brain tissue. In Alzheimer's disease this elimination of protein fragments does not take place. **These fragments accumulate to form hard, insoluble plaques among the glial cells.** This accumulated amyloid is the "bony structures" noted by Dr. Alzheimer. Glial cells comprise 80% of the cell structure of the brain, while neurons make up the other 20%.

Neurofibrillary Tangles

These insoluble twisted fibers are found **inside the neurons** of the brain. These tangles are primarily abnormal **tau protein**. The tau protein becomes abnormal by having a chemical called "phosphate" attached to it in the wrong places by enzymes called "kinases" or by being cut in the wrong way by severing enzymes called "proteases." It is the abnormal tau that accumulates inside the neuron and causes neuronal death. **Tau protein**, in healthy nerve cells helps keep the microtubules of the neurons in the proper position and shape. Microtubules helps in the transport of nutrients and other important substances from one part of the neuron to another part of the neuron. In Alzheimer's and some other types of dementias, however, the tau protein is abnormal and causes the microtubule to collapse. **This stresses the neuron so that it cannot function properly.**

II. Frontotemporal Lobar Degeneration (Dementia) (FTLD)

Frontotemporal Lobar Degeneration (FTLD), another progressive form of dementia, refers to a group of degenerative dementias that share many clinical features, FTLD is the result of progressive damage to cells in the anterior temporal and/or frontal lobes of the brain. The disorders are also known as frontotemporal dementias or Picks disease. The hallmark of FTLD is a gradual, progressive decline in behavior and/or language at an early age onset. As the disease progresses, it becomes increasingly difficult for victim of this disease to plan or organize activities, behave appropriately in social or work settings, interact with others, and care for oneself. This loss of skills result in increasing dependency on their caregiver. The disease progresses to the point that the person eventually loses all the skills for Activities of Daily Living (ADL) and must be cared for 24/7. The onset of FTLD symptoms typically occurs in the 50s to early 60s, but has been seen as early as 21 and as late as 80 years. The average age of onset is about 60 years. FTLD occurs equally in men and women. In a small percentage of cases it is inherited as an Autosomal Dominate genetic disease.

FTLD represents an estimated 5% of all dementia cases and is recognized as one of the **most common dementias affecting a younger population**. It is estimated that FTLD affects approximately 250,000 Americans. While there are currently no treatments to slow or stop the progression of this disease, FTLD research is yielding a greater understanding of the disorders. We anticipate that this knowledge will result in a growing number of potential therapeutics entering clinical testing within the next few years.

Approximately 10% of FTD cases are
Inherited
(50% chance for each child and sibling for
inheriting the gene and developing FTD)

50-70% of FTD cases are
Sporadic
(Not inherited)
Family members have
general population
risk

20-40% of FTD cases are
Familial
(May be inherited)
Family members are at increased,
though undetermined, risk,
probably due to unidentified
susceptibility genes

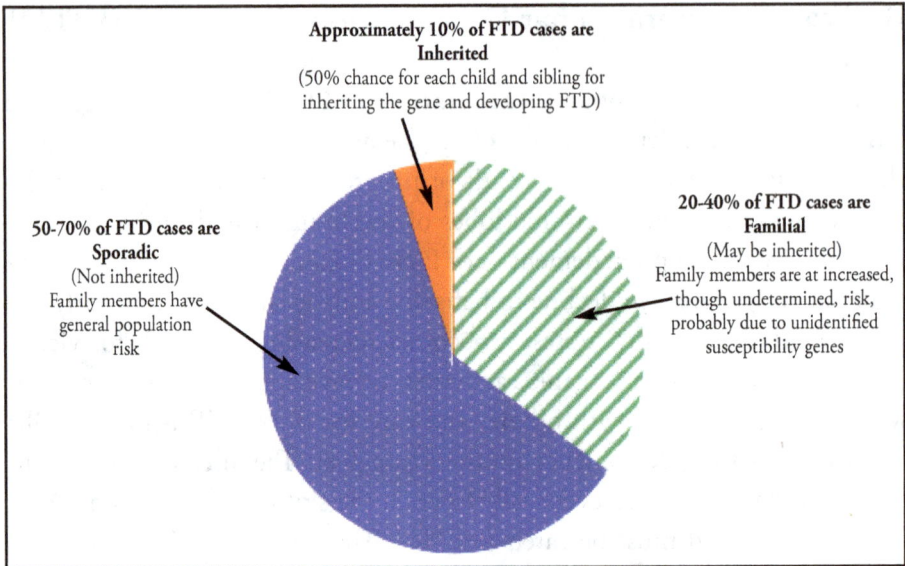

Information obtained from The Association for Frontotemporal Dementia
www.FTD-Picks.org/frontotemporal-dementias/genetics

Types of Frontotemporal Lobular Dementia (FTLD)

- **Behavioral variant FTLD (bvFTLD)**

    Behavioral variant FTLD (bvFTLD) is frontotemporal dementia **characterized by early and progressive changes in personality, emotional blunting, and/or loss of empathy**. It is characterized by difficulty in controlling behavior that often results in inappropriate responses or activities. Impairment of language may also occur but is less prominent and would appear as a word-finding problem. Onset of bvFTLD typically occurs sometime in the 50s, though it can occur as early as age 20 or as late as age 80. As with all FTLDs, the course of bvFTLD will vary from one person to another. Not every symptom will be experienced by every person, nor will these symptoms develop in a prescribed sequence.

- **Corticobasal degeneration (CBD)**

    Corticobasal degeneration (CBD) is a progressive neurological disorder that **may involve the motor system, cognition or both**. Classically, it begins as a movement disorder, with affected individuals showing a unilateral (one sided) paucity of movement, and muscle rigidity with a tremor. **Strength remains normal** but the limb becomes progressively less useful because of the problems with tone, slowness, tremor, and praxis. Praxis (apraxia) is when the strength is adequate to perform a function, but **the patient can't do it because of a "disconnect" between the thought and the action**. Initial symptoms of CBD often begin around age 60 and become bilateral as the disease progresses. A patient with CBD may first present with a language disorder and develop the motor symptoms over time.

Some physicians and investigators use the term "corticobasal syndrome" (CBS) when referring to the clinical symptoms and signs patients experience, and reserve the term CBD for cases which meet neuropathologic criteria. This distinction can be important because some patients with CBS prove to have other neuropathological diagnoses. Alternatively, there are sometimes unusual clinical symptoms in patients with pathological features of CBD.

- **FTLD-Motor Neuron Disease (MND).**

    Researchers have begun to recognize **an important connection between frontotemporal dementia (FTLD) and amyotrophic lateral sclerosis (ALS, or Lou Gehrig's disease)**. FTLD is a syndrome of progressive changes in behavior and language due to loss of function of neurons in the frontal and temporal lobes. Usually, FTLD has relatively little effect on the parts of the nervous system that control movement, and so many FTLD patients remain physically strong and relatively agile until late in the illness. However, in about 10-15% of patients with FTLD, the disease also involves the nerve cells controlling voluntary movement, called motor neurons. When this occurs, the syndrome is called FTLD with motor neuron disease (FTLD/MND).

    Patients with FTLD/MND may present with the same behavioral and/or language changes seen in other subtypes of FTLD. In this syndrome, however, these changes are accompanied by a deterioration of motor neurons that **manifest as weakness in the muscles** with stiffness, difficulty making fine movements, atrophy (shrinkage) of the muscles, and fine muscle twitches and cramps. Muscle changes can affect the arms and/or legs on one or both sides of the body or the face, tongue, and mouth, depending on how the nervous system is affected in that individual.

As the disease worsens, more parts of the motor system become involved.

Patients with FTLD/MND may first present with features of either FTLD or ALS with the additional symptoms developing as the disease progresses. All patients with FTLD/MND will experience a gradual, steady decline in functioning.

- **Pick's Disease (PICKS)**

    Pick's Disease (PICKS) is the original term for frontotemporal dementia characterized by a slowly **progressive deterioration of social skills and changes in personality, or with impairment of language**. Currently, the term Pick's Disease is reserved for a specific pathology with Pick Bodies, which are abnormal collections of the protein tau in the brain. A diagnosis of Pick's disease can only be confirmed through postmortem examination of brain tissue.

    Clinically, it may be indistinguishable from the behavioral, aphasic, or Parkinson-like presentations of FTLD. Onset typically occurs sometime in the 50s, though it can occur as early as age 20 or as late as age 80. As with all FTLDs, the course of Pick's Disease will vary from one person to another. Not every symptom will be experienced by every person, nor will these symptoms develop in a prescribed sequence.

- **Progressive Aphasia**

    Progressive Aphasia, also known as **Progressive Nonfluent Aphasia (PNFA)**, is a language disorder separate from aphasia resulting after a stroke. It is also called **Primary Progressive Aphasia (PPA)** or **Agrammatic Aphasia** and is reviewed here. Some consider Semantic Dementia a progressive aphasia, and it is reviewed separately.

    The presenting feature in people with PNFA is a **deterioration in their ability to produce speech**. These patients first become hesitant in their speech, begin to talk less, and eventually become mute. Current research suggests that the fundamental loss in PNFA is a deterioration in knowledge of the grammatical organization and the production of sounds for language.

    Unlike other FTLD subtypes, PNFA generally does not produce changes in behavior or personality until later stages of the disease. Most people with progressive aphasia maintain the ability to care for themselves, keep up outside interests and, in some instances, remain employed for a few years after onset of the disorder.

- **Semantic dementia (SD)**

  Semantic dementia (SD) is a disorder of language in which patients demonstrate a progressive deterioration of understanding words, especially nouns, and recognizing objects, while other cognitive faculties remain remarkably spared. Specifically, patients with SD **retain the ability to produce fluent speech, but without key words, this speech becomes increasing difficult to understand. SD patients also lose the ability to recognize the meaning of specific words, or to spontaneously name familiar, everyday objects**. As with all FTLDs, as the disorder progresses and the primary symptoms (in the case of SD, language deficits) worsen, the patient may also develop other FTLD features, including behavioral, social, or motor difficulties.

- **Progressive supranuclear palsy (PSP)**

  Progressive supranuclear palsy (PSP)is a rare brain disorder that causes serious and permanent problems with **control of gait and balance**. PSP is a **visual disturbance**, which results from a **progressive inability to coordinate eye movements**. PSP is related to both Parkinson's disease and FTLD.

  Additional motor symptoms similar to those seen in Parkinson's disease and other features of frontotemporal dementia, such as behavioral and social dysfunction and cognitive decline, may develop. Depression and apathy are common mood symptoms. **PSP is not itself life-threatening**.

III. Dementia with Lewy Bodies (DLB)

The information below is taken from the following website and can be referred to in its entirety at:
www.ninds.nih.gov/disorders/dementiawithlewybodies/dementiawithlewybodies.htm

Caregivers of a loved one with Lewy Body Dementia are aware of **three characteristics** exhibited by individuals of this progressive dementia. The victims of this disease have **large fluctuations in alertness and attention**. They have **periods of drowsiness, lethargy, catatonic episodes, and disorganized speech**. A hallmark of DLB patients is that they have recurrent **visual hallucinations**, and they exhibit **parkinsonian motor skill difficulties**. Another characteristic of DLB cases is that they suffer from **rigidity and loss of spontaneous movement**. Additionally, DLB patients **often are depressed**.

Scientist attribute DLB to a build up of bits of alpha-synuclein protein bodies (Lewy Bodies), inside the nuclei of neurons in the brain. The accumulation of these Lewy Bodies in the areas of brain that control memories and motor control skills are the cause and affect of how these individuals interact. Alpha-synuclein accumulations are also found in Parkinson's disease, multisystem atrophy, and other "synucleinopathies." Lewy bodies are also found in some Alzheimer's patients. Some neurologists have even suggested that it might be conceivable that a patient might have DLB and Alzheimer's disease concurrently.

As with the other progressive dementias, there is no cure for DLB. Drug treatments for DLB patients are aimed at controlling the cognitive, psychiatric, and motor symptoms disorders. Acetylcholinesterase inhibitors, such as donepezil and rivastigmine, are primarily used to treat the cognitive symptoms. But the use of drugs may also be of some benefit in reducing the psychiatric and motor symptoms. Many physicians tend to avoid giving antipsychotics for the hallucinatory symptoms of DLB because of the risk that neuroleptic sensitivity to the drug could worsen the motor symptoms. Some individuals with DLB may benefit from the use of levodopa for their rigidity and loss of spontaneous movement.

Life expectancy after diagnosis is about eight (8) years. ❖

Chapter 10

The Science

Many caregivers have a need to understand what is causing their loved one's difficulties, but they do not have a reference point from which to begin to understand. This section starts from the beginning by explaining the basic components and leads to the basics of life: protein, DNA, RNA, and more. It takes you from the smallest entity known to DNA.

How things are made

1. Quarks (the smallest entity known)
2. Protons, Neutrons, and Electrons
3. The 118 known elements
4. Organic Compounds
5. Amino Acids
6. Protein
7. The Cell
   (a) Structural Proteins (Polypetides Chains that form cell walls)
   (b) Chemical Proteins for special cell and intracellar functions
   (c) DNA, RNA, and mRNA.
      i. Genes
         A. Autosomal Dominant
         B. Autosomal Recessive
      ii. Chromosomes

Quarks are the building blocks of Protons, Neutrons, and Electrons

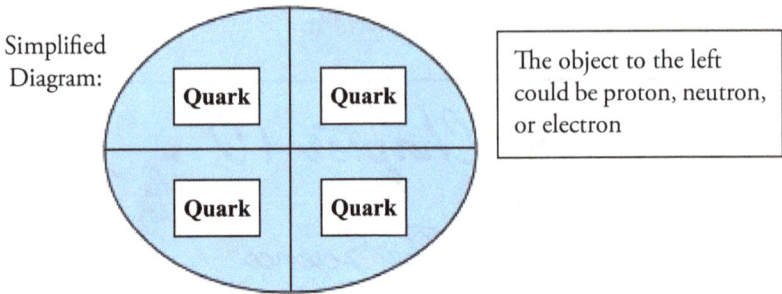

Simplified Diagram:

Quark	Quark
Quark	Quark

The object to the left could be proton, neutron, or electron

All of the elements are composed of even smaller components called sub-atomic particles. These sub-atomic particles are protons, neutrons, and electrons. Sub-atomic particles are made up of the smallest known particles called "**quarks.**" There are six different types of quarks that are the sub-structure of Protons, Neutrons, and Electrons, which are the building blocks of the Atomic Elements.

Shown in the **Periodic Table** that follows are the atomic elements, which are the building blocks of all "matter" as we know it. This Periodic Chart provides scientists a great deal of information about each element.

Elements are the building blocks of everything in our universe, even us. Many of these are common elements and may be purchased when visiting the Health and Nutrition stores. For example:

12. (Mg) Magnesium
26. (Fe) Iron
28. (Ni) Nickel
29. (Cu) Copper
30. (Zn) Zinc
11. (Na) Sodium

19. (K) Potassium
20. (Ca) Calcium
24. (Cr) Chromium
47. (Ag) Silver
79. (Au) Gold (Ag)

I am sure you could find even more with close inspection.

Deciphering the chart: 1 = the atomic number, (H) = the abbreviation of Hydrogen. The chart is designed with the smallest atomic numbered element (hydrogen), and progresses to the largest atomic element (Uuo 118) with the largest number of protons, electrons, and neutrons.

Periodic Chart of the Elements

Group→ ↓Period	1	2	3	4	5	6	7	8	9	10	11	12	13	14	15	16	17	18
1	1 H																	2 He
2	3 Li	4 Be											5 B	6 C	7 N	8 O	9 F	10 Ne
3	11 Na	12 Mg											13 Al	14 Si	15 P	16 S	17 Cl	18 Ar
4	19 K	20 Ca	21 Sc	22 Ti	23 V	24 Cr	25 Mn	26 Fe	27 Co	28 Ni	29 Cu	30 Zn	31 Ga	32 Ge	33 As	34 Se	35 Br	36 Kr
5	37 Rb	38 Sr	39 Y	40 Zr	41 Nb	42 Mo	43 Tc	44 Ru	45 Rh	46 Pd	47 Ag	48 Cd	49 In	50 Sn	51 Sb	52 Te	53 I	54 Xe
6	55 Cs	56 Ba		72 Hf	73 Ta	74 W	75 Re	76 Os	77 Ir	78 Pt	79 Au	80 Hg	81 Tl	82 Pb	83 Bi	84 Po	85 At	86 Rn
7	87 Fr	88 Ra		104 Rf	105 Db	106 Sg	107 Bh	108 Hs	109 Mt	110 Ds	111 Rg	112 Uub	113 Uut	114 Uuq	115 Uup	116 Uuh	117 Uus	118 Uuo

Lanthanides	57 La	58 Ce	59 Pr	60 Nd	61 Pm	62 Sm	63 Eu	64 Gd	65 Tb	66 Dy	67 Ho	68 Er	69 Tm	70 Yb	71 Lu
Actinides	89 Ac	90 Th	91 Pa	92 U	93 Np	94 Pu	95 Am	96 Cm	97 Bk	98 Cf	99 Es	100 Fm	101 Md	102 No	103 Lr

A List of Elements :

The number is the Atomic number of the Element, the ( ) is elements symbol, and the name follows the associated number and symbol. The elements are listed numerically from the most simple, 1: (H) Hydrogen, to the most complex, 118: (Uuo) unknown.

1: (H) Hydrogen
2: (He) Helium
3: (Li) Lithium
4: (Be) Beryllium
5: (B) Boron
6: (C) Carbon
7: (N) Nitrogen
8: (O) Oxygen
9: (F) Fluorine
10: (Ne) Neon
11: (Na) Sodium
12: (Mg) Magnesium
13: (Al) Aluminum
14: (Si)Silicon
15: (P) Phosphorus
16: (S) Sulfur
17: (Cl) Chlorine
18: (Ar) Argon
19: (K) Potassium
20: (Ca) Calcium
21: (Sc) Scandium
22: (T) Titanium

23: (V) Vanadium
24: (Cr) Chromium
25: (Mn) Manganese
26: (Fe) Iron
27: (Co) Cobalt
28: (Ni) Nickel
29: (Cu) Copper
30: (Zn) Zinc
31: (Ga) Galium
32: (Gm) Germanium
33: (As) Arsenic
34: (Se) Selenium
35: (Br) Bromide
36: (Kr) Krypton
37: (Rb) Rubidium
38: (Sr) Strontium
39: (Y) Yttrium
40: (Zr) Zirconium
41: (Nb) Niobium
42: (Mo) Molybdenum
43: (Tc) Technetium
44: (Ru) Ruthenium

45: (Rh) Rhodium
46: (Pd) Palladium
47: (Ag) Silver
48: (Cd) Cadmium
49: (In) Indium
50: (Sn) Tin
51: (Sb) Antimony
52: (Te) Tellurium
53: (I) Iodine
54: (Xe) Xenon
55: (Cs) Caesium
56: (Ba) Barium
57: (La) Lanthanum
58: (Ce) Cerium
59: (Pr) Praseodymium
60: (Nd) Neodymium
61: (Pm) Promethium
62: (Sm) Samarium
63: (Eu) Europeium
64: (Gd) Gadolinium
65: (Tb) Terbium
66: (Dy) Dysprosium

67: (Ho) Holmium
68: (Er) Erbium
69: (Tm) Thulium
70: (Yb) Ytterbium
71: (Lu) Lutetium
72: (Hf) Hafrium
73: (Ta) Tantalum
74: (W) Tungsten
75: (Re) Rhenium
76: (Os) Osmium
77: (Ir) Iridium
78: (Pt) Platinium
79: (Au) Gold
80: (Hg) Mercury
81: (Tl) Thallium
82: (Pb) Lead
83: (Bi) Bismuth
84: (Po) Polonium
85: (At) Astatine
86: (Rn) Radon ....
118: (Uuo) (unknown)

The element **Helium** is the **most basic element** with all three of the subatomic components, with one proton, one neutron, and one electron.

The simplest element in the universe is hydrogen. It has one proton and one electron, but no neutron. Hydrogen, with its chemical cousin helium, comprises 99% of the known universe.

As we study the Periodic Chart, there are things that are easily recognizable to us, and many come in combinations that we understand because of our daily use of these elements. When there are combinations of elements, we call them molecules.

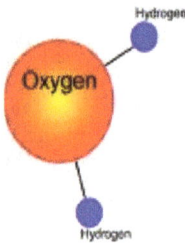

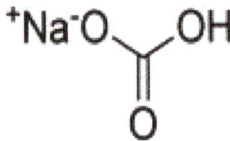

Water molecule (H_2O)   Baking Soda (NaO_3H)   Table Salt (NaCl)

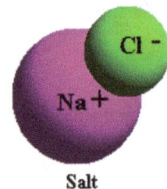

Organic Chemistry is a special group of elements comprised of hydrogen (H), carbon (C), oxygen (O), nitrogen (N), sulfur (S), and phosphorus (P), and a group called the "halogen group" (floride, chloride, bromide, and iodide). It is this special group of hydro-carbons and their multiple combinations that are the building blocks of all life forms.

Nitrogen is a significant building block for proteins. Nitrogen is also the **most dominant** element in the atmosphere, contributing to 78% of the air, whereas oxygen comprises 21%. We get ammonia (NH_4) during the process of lightning going through the air and fusing the nitrogen with hydrogen. The ammonia (NH_4) that is produced goes into the soil as fertilizer. In addition, nitrogen when combined with the other organic elements forms **amino acids. The 20 known amino acid groups are the building blocks of proteins** for cell wall construction and other vital cell functions.

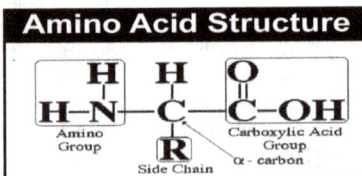

Amino Acid Structure

Diagram of a basic amino acid, which is defined by the "amino (NH_2) protein group"

90

We exist because these basic molecules, compounds, and proteins combine to make us into a living entity. We, as organisms, are 98% water and a plethora of compounds and proteins.

Some of the more recognizable organic compounds are water, carbon dioxide, an unlimited number of proteins that produce, for example, sugars and hormones. Almost everything that happens in our bodies is due to the interaction of chemical compounds. For example, calcium (Ca) assists us with blood coagulation … and sodium and potassium help with the synaptic process of the chemical communication by neurons in the brain. Iron (Fe) is essential for oxygen/carbon dioxide transfer in respiration.

Proteins

The National Institute of Medical Sciences does a wonderful job of explaining **"proteins"** and their functions. Proteins are the "worker molecules" within the body that are necessary, not only to brain activity, but to every activity in the body. **Proteins are the KEY components of all living things.**

Note the explanation below, taken directly from The National Institute of General Medical Science's website:

Proteins are like long necklaces with differently shaped beads. Each "bead" is a small molecule called an amino acid. There are 20 standard amino acids, each with its own shape, size, and properties.

Proteins typically contain from 50 to 2,000 amino acids hooked end-to-end in many combinations. Each protein has its own sequence of amino acids.

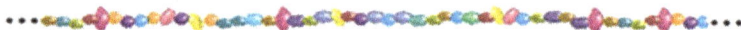

Proteins are made of amino acids hooked end-to-end like beads on a necklace.

These amino acid chains do not remain straight and orderly. They must twist and fold into their final, or "native," conformation. They buckle, folding in upon themselves, the knobs of some amino acids nestling into grooves in others.

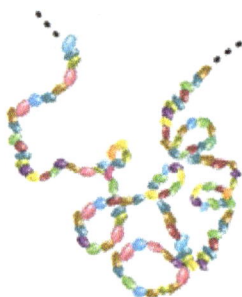

The final shape enables proteins to accomplish their function in your body.

This process is complete almost immediately after proteins are made. Most proteins fold in less than a second, although the largest and most complex proteins may require several seconds to fold. Most proteins need help from other proteins, called "chaperones," to fold efficiently.

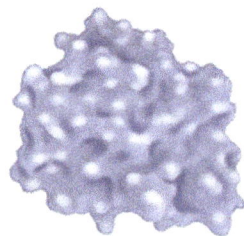

When these "necklaces" fold and twist, they create different proteins, which have unique tasks to accomplish. Some proteins have the job of regulating the genetic material (DNA), some, the enzymes that facilitate the chemical reactions necessary for normal activity in the brain and elsewhere. This folding is believed to be encoded in the sequence of the amino acids. The miss-folding of the proteins, scientists call "the protein folding problem." The long and short of it is, when an amino acid has miss-folded, an error (or mutation) occurs and disease results.

Proteins have many different functions in our bodies. By studying the structures of proteins, we are better able to understand how they function normally and how some proteins with abnormal shapes can cause disease.

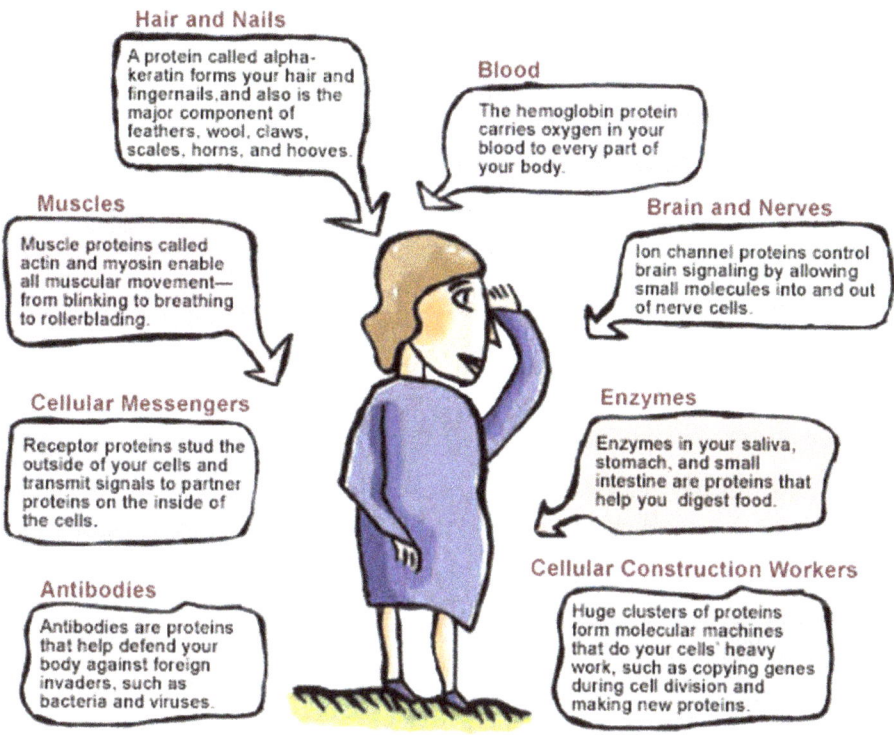

Hair and Nails

A protein called alpha-keratin forms your hair and fingernails,and also is the major component of feathers, wool, claws, scales, horns, and hooves.

Blood

The hemoglobin protein carries oxygen in your blood to every part of your body.

Muscles

Muscle proteins called actin and myosin enable all muscular movement—from blinking to breathing to rollerblading.

Brain and Nerves

Ion channel proteins control brain signaling by allowing small molecules into and out of nerve cells.

Cellular Messengers

Receptor proteins stud the outside of your cells and transmit signals to partner proteins on the inside of the cells.

Enzymes

Enzymes in your saliva, stomach, and small intestine are proteins that help you digest food.

Antibodies

Antibodies are proteins that help defend your body against foreign invaders, such as bacteria and viruses.

Cellular Construction Workers

Huge clusters of proteins form molecular machines that do your cells' heavy work, such as copying genes during cell division and making new proteins.

Source: National Institute of General Medical Sciences, The Structures of Life.

The Cell

The cell gives organization to functions that need to be accomplished for the cell and for the tissue that the cell is a part of or supports. Each sub-structure has a specific purpose to accomplish and specific tasks as defined in the "Glossary of Animal Cell Terms" on the next page.

In a simplified analysis, this is what happens with cell metabolism. The nucleoli and nucleus send information and commands into the cytoplasm for the manufacture of proteins. This mechanism is accomplished through tRNA. tRna is basically a message: **"'Make something' with the instructions that I am giving you**," as defined by the DNA in the chromosomes. This message is received by ribosomes, which are in essence manufacturing sites. The ribosome follows the instructions sent from the nucleus via the tRNA. 90% or more of what is manufactured is a vast array of proteins that will support the life of the cell or tissue. Some of those proteins are enzymes, some are lipids, hormones, and steroids. The list of proteins to be manufactured are innumerable.

One of the sub-cellular components are the vacuoles that act as "trash cans" to take unused, unusable, or defectively made protein to the cell membrane where the vacuole can dump the unwanted material out into the intra-cellular cavities or space.

It is believed by some scientists that the accumulated, faulty tau protein, Lewy bodies, Pick bodies, and chromatin bodies may simply be excess faulty proteins that the vacuoles cannot identify and process for "dumping." Thus, these bodies accumulate in excess to the point that they become toxic and kill the cell. This concept is one of many being proposed as to how the neurons are killed at an accelerated rate in these dementias.

Protein Manufacturing in The Animal (Human) Cell

Proteins, including faulty proteins, are manufactured in the "smooth endoplasmic reticulum" (Smooth ER), the sub-cellular portion of the animal cell.

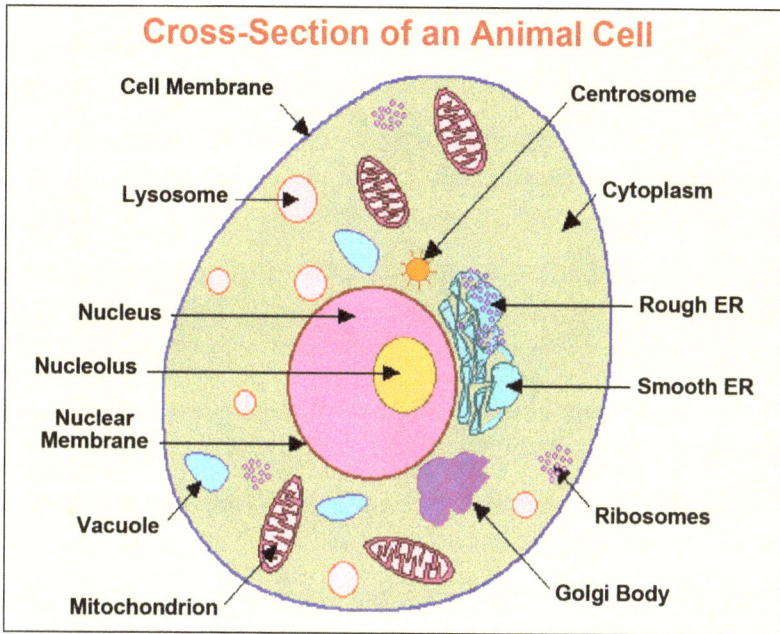

Cross-Section of an Animal Cell

Glossary of "Animal Cell" Terms

For clarity, we have added an analogy in blue after each definition.

cell membrane – the thin layer of protein and fat that surrounds the cell. The cell membrane is semi-permeable, allowing some substances to pass into the cell and blocking others. **The cell membrane is the outside of the factory walls. It has doors and windows (pores) that will allow things to go in or out when it is appropriate.**

centrosome – (also called the "microtubule organizing center") a small body located near the nucleus. It has a dense center and radiating tubules. The centrosome is where microtubules are made. During cell division (mitosis), the centrosome divides and the two parts move to opposite sides of the dividing cell. The centriole is the dense center of the centrosome. **The centrosome is like the vacuum tubes at banks that send packages of information from one part of the cell to another.**

cytoplasm – the jellylike material outside the cell nucleus in which the organelles are located. **The cytoplasm of our factory is the air within the walls.**

Golgi body – (also called the Golgi apparatus or Golgi complex) a flattened, layered, sac-like organelle that looks like a stack of pancakes and is located near the nucleus. It produces the membranes that surround the lysosomes. The Golgi body packages proteins and carbohydrates into membrane-bound vesicles for "export" from the cell. **The golgi complex are the "trash compactors" that prepare waste material to be taken out of the factory.**

lysosome – (also called cell vesicles) spherical organelles surrounded by a membrane; they contain digestive enzymes. This is where the digestion of cell nutrients takes place. **These are the cans of solvents used to dissolve things in the factory.**

mitochondrion – spherical to rod-shaped organelles with a double membrane. The inner membrane is infolded many times, forming a series of projections (called cristae). The mitochondrion converts the energy stored in glucose into ATP (adenosine triphosphate) for the cell. **This is the air-handling structure of the factory. It also produces a lot of heat when it is needed (respiration).**

nuclear membrane – the membrane that surrounds the nucleus. **This is the wall to the "office" of our factory.**

nucleolus – an organelle within the nucleus - it is where ribosomal RNA is produced. Some cells have more than one nucleolus. **This is the marketing department for our factory.**

nucleus – spherical body containing many organelles, including the nucleolus. The nucleus controls many of the functions of the cell (by controlling protein synthesis) and contains DNA (in chromosomes). The nucleus is surrounded by the nuclear membrane. **This is the conference room where the owners or board of directors meet to makes business plans.**

ribosome – small organelles composed of RNA-rich cytoplasmic granules that are sites of protein synthesis. **This part of the plant is where the employees are making product to be used in the factory.**

rough endoplasmic reticulum – (rough ER) a vast system of interconnected, membranous, infolded and convoluted sacks that are located in the cell's cytoplasm (the ER is continuous with the outer nuclear membrane). Rough ER is covered with ribosomes that give it a rough appearance. Rough ER transports materials through the cell and produces proteins in sacks called cisternae (which are sent to the Golgi body, or inserted into the cell membrane). **This is where packets of product are made for distribution to the Golgi or for use in the factory walls (cell membrane).**

smooth endoplasmic reticulum – (smooth ER) a vast system of interconnected, membranous, infolded and convoluted tubes that are located in the cell's cytoplasm (the ER is continuous with the outer nuclear membrane). The space within the ER is called the ER lumen. Smooth ER transports materials through the cell. It contains enzymes and produces and digests lipids (fats) and membrane proteins; smooth ER buds off from rough ER, moving the newly-made proteins and lipids to the Golgi body, lysosomes, and membranes **Smooth ER is a transport system for many products that were made and need to go to specific areas in the factory.**

vacuole – fluid-filled, membrane-surrounded cavities inside a cell. The vacuole fills with food being digested and waste material that is on its way out of the cell. **These are the trash cans produced by the Golgi trash compactors. These vacuoles will move the trash to the outside walls of the factory, where doors or windows will open in the factory wall to flush the waste out of the building.**

The cell continues the life process by duplicating and replicating DNA and RNA.

Genes

The following is from the AFTD website:

Genes are specific subunits or groups of DNA along the chromosomes. Just as our chromosomes come in pairs, so do our genes. Most genes code for proteins (or chemicals) that have a specific function in the body.

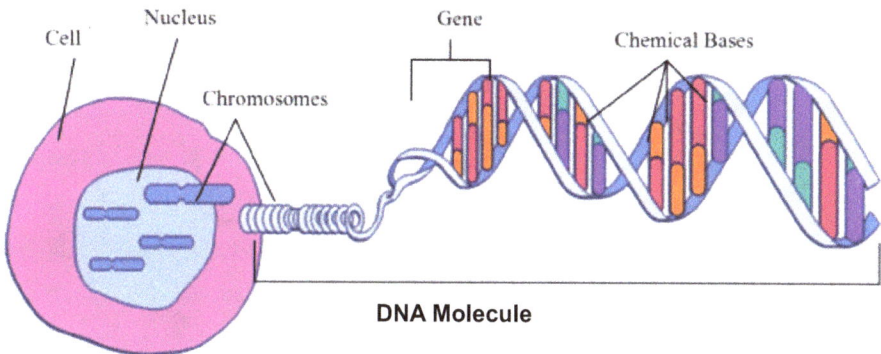

DNA Molecule

The following analogy may be helpful: One can think of a gene as a long word. Every letter in the word is a piece of DNA. Just like words, genes must be correctly "spelled," or have the correct DNA code in order to function properly.

There are two types of "misspellings" that can occur in our DNA.

One type includes words with **multiple spellings but with the same meaning**, or a misspelling that is silent and allows the word to still be read correctly. For example, the word "theater" is sometimes spelled as "theatre." Despite this alteration, you still understand the word and its meaning. This type of alteration in the DNA code is called a "**polymorphism**." The body can continue to function normally when there is a polymorphism.

The second type of misspelling involves **changes to the word that alter the meaning or make the word unreadable**. An example is if the word "good" were changed to "god." One would not be able to make sense out of "good." This type of misspelling or change in the DNA code is called a "**mutation**." Mutations alter the function of the gene and are often associated with disease.

Inherited Conditions

Inherited conditions can be passed on (inherited) in families in different ways.

Autosomal Dominant Conditions

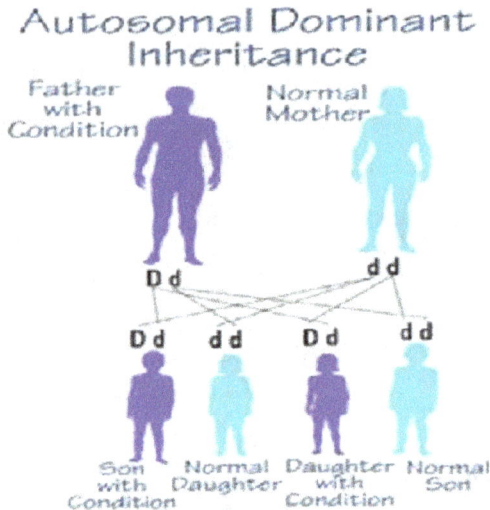

Autosomal Dominant Inheritance

Autosomal dominant conditions affect males and females equally, and only one gene of the pair needs to be abnormal for the individual to have the condition. Every child of an individual with an autosomal dominant condition has a 50% chance of inheriting the mutation and having the disorder (Huntington's disease and achondroplasia, a common form of dwarfism, are examples of autosomal dominant conditions). When examining a family history for an autosomal dominant condition, oftentimes one will identify multiple individuals in each generation with the condition. It is important to understand that **if an individual did not inherit the abnormal gene then he/she cannot pass it on**.

Autosomal recessive conditions affect males and females equally, but **both** copies of the disease gene need to be abnormal for the individual to have the condition. Autosomal recessive conditions can be passed on when each parent is a "carrier" for the condition, and their offspring have a 25% risk of inheriting the condition. "Carriers" have one abnormal copy of the gene but do not have clinical symptoms and **are not at increased risk to develop the condition**. A family history of a recessive condition can reveal multiple individuals in a single generation (brothers and sisters) with the condition; in the case of small families, however, there may be only one affected individual. Autosomal recessive conditions also appear more frequently among individuals with the same ethnic background or among individuals who marry within the same family. (Sickle cell anemia and cystic fibrosis are examples of autosomal recessive conditions.)

Other types of inheritance include conditions that are linked to the sex chromosomes (X-linked) or those that are only passed on through maternal transmission. Neither of these patterns has been identified in the inheritance of FTLDs. Features of Autosomal Dominant Inheritance: The condition appears in multiple individuals in multiple generations, and each affected individual has an affected parent. Any offspring of an affected parent has a 50% risk of inheriting the condition. Non-affected individuals do not transmit the condition to offspring. Males and females are equally likely to have the condition.

Features of Autosomal Recessive Inheritance

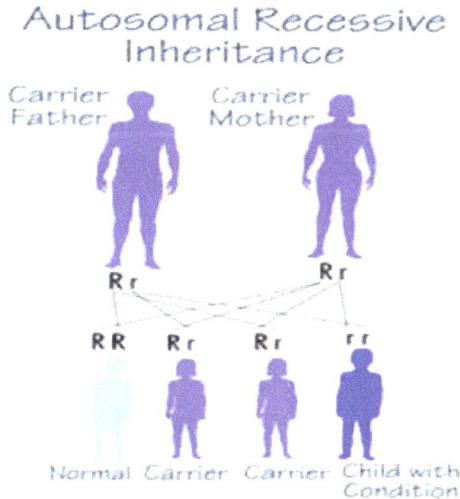

Autosomal Recessive Inheritance

Carrier Father
Carrier Mother

R r
R r

R R   R r   R r   r r

Normal Carrier Carrier Child with Condition

The condition appears in multiple members of a siblingship, not in the parents or offspring. If the family is small there may only be one affected individual. The recurrence risk for each sibling is 25%. Males and females are equally likely to have the condition. Parents may be consanguineous (related by blood).

Based on genetic research, we now appreciate that when one examines the family tree, not all "genetic conditions" show a clear pattern of inheritance. This is because not all are caused by a single gene. Rather, many conditions, especially neurodegenerative conditions, are caused by changes in multiple genes that create a susceptibility, or increased risk, for the condition. When individuals with this increased risk encounter an additional environmental influence, e.g., head trauma or infection, the medical condition then appears. Conditions that are caused by both genetic and environmental influences are called "multifactorial."

Often, multifactorial conditions are seen in multiple family members but without a specific pattern to the inheritance. Thus, another term used for these conditions is "**familial.**"

The specific base-pairing of DNA aids in reproduction of the double helix when more genetic material is needed (such as during reproduction, to pass on characteristics from parent to offspring).

Within this coil of DNA lies all the information needed to produce everything in the human body. A strand of DNA may be millions, or billions, of base-pairs long. Different segments of the DNA molecule code for different characteristics in the body. A **Gene** is a relatively small segment of DNA that codes for the synthesis of a specific protein. This protein then will play a structural or functional role in the body. A **chromosome** is a larger collection of DNA that contains many genes and the support proteins needed to control these genes.

The ABCs of DNA

How "Spelling" Mistakes Can Result in Faulty Proteins

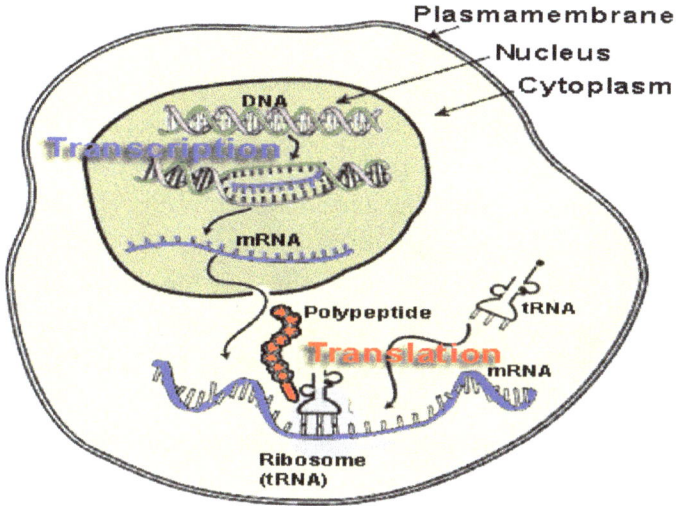

Dr. Gail V.W. Johnson, University of Rochester, has graciously contributed the following article on the ABCs of DNA and how faulty proteins contribute to the cause of dementia.

Almost everyone has heard about "DNA," but what is it? How does it work, and what goes wrong in "genetic" diseases?

The cell is the basic building block of all living organisms, and humans are multi-cellular organisms, made up of trillions of cells. The majority of cells in the human body contain a structure called a "nucleus," which is the data center. The nucleus contains the information that the cell needs to orchestrate the development and life of the body. Contained in the nucleus are structures called "chromosomes." Humans have 23 pairs of chromosomes. Chromosomes are made up of DNA molecules in complex with a variety of proteins, such as histones. Although the proteins of the chromosomes play important structural and regulatory roles, it is the DNA that contains the code of life.

DNA is the abbreviation for deoxyribonucleic acid, which is the genetic material present in the cells of all living organisms. DNA is the fundamental building block for an individual's entire genetic makeup. A person's DNA is

101

the same in every cell (with a nucleus). The DNA in a person's blood is the same as the DNA in their brain, muscles, and skin cells. The DNA is the instruction manual for the cell; it provides all the information the cell needs to make and maintain itself. Chemically, DNA consists of two long strands of simple building blocks called "nucleotides" in a structure that resembles a twisted ladder and is often called a "double helix." The "sides" of this ladder structure are made up of sugars and phosphate groups held together by strong bonds. The sides of these ladders have direction (like a sentence) and run in opposite directions to each other and are therefore anti-parallel to each other. The "rungs" of this DNA ladder are molecules called "bases" and are attached to the sugars of the sides of the ladder. There are four bases, and it is the order of these bases that spell out the instruction manual of the cell. The four bases that are found in every human DNA molecule are (A) adenine, (G) guanine—which is purines, (C) cytosine, and (T) thymine—which are pyrimidines. These bases are attached to the sides of the ladder and project towards and interact with each other to form the rungs of the structure. They also interact in a specific way to form a base pair, "A" always binds to "T," and "G" always binds to "C." A sequence of three bases, e.g., CAG, is the essential informational unit called a "codon," and it "spells" the information needed to eventually make a protein (how this happens is described below). Because the strands or sides of the ladder are anti parallel, one strand would read "CAG"—this is the sense strand, while the reverse (or antisense) strand would read GTC. The sequence of bases spells the genetic code of life.

The next question is, "How is the genetic code maintained?" Most cells divide to make new cells **(although brain cells, also called "neurons," do NOT divide, which means that they must repair when injured because they will not be replaced by a new cell)**. When a cell divides, it must replicate its DNA so that the two daughter cells have the same genetic information as their parent. To do this, the two strands, or sides, of the DNA separate, and then each strand's complementary DNA sequence is recreated by enzymes that bring in the correct complementary base (e.g., when there is a "T," the enzyme brings an "A" to form the base pairs of the intact DNA, or double helix. In this way, both daughter cells end up with identical DNA.

The purpose of DNA is to provide all information needed to make all the proteins in the cell, which in essence *is* the cell. The first step in this process is called "transcription" and is the primary function of ribonucleic acid (RNA). RNA is similar to DNA in that it is made up of sugar, phosphate, and bases. But there are also differences. First, RNA is usually just one strand, instead of the double-stranded DNA. Also, RNA does not contain the base thymine but, rather, contains Uracil (U), which then compliments with adenine (A). In the process of transcription, specific stretches of DNA that carry the codes to make specific proteins are "copied" onto the messenger RNA (mRNA). In this process, the DNA strands separate in certain areas, and a copy is made of just this area using the strands by a large group of proteins, with the central one being called "RNA polymerase." Base matches are made in a manner similar to when DNA was replicated. "C" and "G" compliment, while "A" compliments to "U." The RNA polymerase complex knows to stop when it gets to what is called a stop codon (the three "words" for stop are TAA, TGA, or TAG). Once transcription of mRNA reaches one of these stop codons it means all the information to make a specific protein is encoded in that mRNA, so the process stops and the mRNA moves out of the nucleus in the cytoplasm of the cell where it will be used to make the protein.

Each mRNA carries the information from a specific portion of the genetic code that is the information needed by the cell to make specific protein. This process of using the mRNA to make a protein is called "translation." The mRNA sequence serves as a template to guide the synthesis of a chain of amino acids to form a specific protein. Once the mRNA is out of the nucleus, it then binds an organelle in the cytoplasm where the protein will be made. The process of translating the information encoded in the mRNA into a protein involves molecules called "transfer RNA" (tRNA). There are many different tRNAs, and each one has a specific unit called an "anti-codon," made up of three nucleotides that compliment the three bases of the codon on the mRNA. For example, if the sequence of the bases in the mRNA were "CAG," the anticodon of the tRNA would be "GUC." In addition, each tRNA contains the amino acid that corresponds to that codon (and there are 20 different amino acids found in the proteins of the human body). For example, the tRNA that has the anticodon, "GUC," also is bound to the amino acid, glutamine. The tRNAs then facilitate the building of the protein by bringing the correct amino acids to be joined together on the ribosome to make a stretch of amino acids (called a "polypeptide") that then goes on to form the protein. The sequence of amino acids is what determines each specific protein. These proteins then go on to perform all the essential functions of the cell. They make the basic structure of the cell (e.g., actin, tubulin, neurofilaments), and they are the enzymes that make energy (e.g., pyruvate dehydrogenase, ATP synthase). Proteins are basically the essence of life. So what happens if a "mistake" occurs in the DNA?

There are many different kinds of "genetic diseases." What will be discussed here is called "inherited autosomal dominant diseases" and in particular when one base is changed. This can happen when a "mistake" is made when the DNA is being copied, and let's say that for some reason there is a mismatch in the pairing of a single base. These are called "point mutations." The cell is actually very good at preventing and correcting mistakes ... but on rare occasions the mistake is not corrected. However, not all "mistakes" are a problem. Many changes in the base pairs of the DNA do not result in changes in the amino acids because there are multiple spellings for each amino acid. In addition, even if the amino acid is changed, it often does not affect the function of the proteins. Additionally, in order for these mutations to be passed on to offspring, they must occur in the sperm or the egg cells. Once the change occurs, however, the cell that maintains that mistake as the "correct" information faithfully copies it. If this mutation is in the sperm or egg, it will be transmitted to the offspring. This becomes a problem when the point mutation in the DNA results in an amino acid change in the protein that makes the protein not do its job correctly and/or take on a new, but toxic, function, which eventually makes the cell sick. This is when a disease will develop. The term "autosomal dominant" means if you get one copy of the mutated DNA (which would come from just one of the parents), you will get the disease.

An example of a family of autosomal dominant diseases is Frontotemporal Dementia linked to Chromosome 17 (FTDP-17). These diseases result from different point mutations, many of which result in single amino acid changes in the protein called "tau." Tau is protein found mostly in nerve cells and is essential to the proper structure and functioning of the nerve cells. These FTDP-17 cause changes in tau that allow it to function at some level for many years; in addition, the cell also has coping strategies to compensate for the impaired tau. However, the nerve cell losing its ability to function and eventually dying occurs mostly in the nerve cells of the front part of the brain. Currently, there is no cure for this disease. However, much effort is being put forth to figure out a way to treat the disease and slow the process down or even stop it. ❖

A word from the author:

As of March 2009, there were 453 gene mutations (mistakes or misspellings of how proteins are made) that contribute or cause the various dementias. Refer to page 97 to find the explanation of these gene mutations.

My family has for 40 years been searching to name the disease they termed "going off." For us, "going off" is an R406W gene mutation of a faulty tau protein. This book is about the monster that has devoured so many members of this family. It is the story of one faulty gene mutation (one of 453). Some scientists believe this monster may have come into existence as far back as the 14th century in Scotland, Ireland, or Wales.

*The website shown below is titled *Alzheimer's Disease and Frontotemporal Dementia Mutation (Gene) Database.* The site is physically located in Belgium, so it may be necessary to select "English" in your browser to have in translated.

*www.molgen.ua.ac.be/ADMutations/default.cfm?MT=0&ML=0&Page=Home

About Faulty Proteins

There are seven (7) groups of faulty proteins that comprise the 453 gene mutations found on the Alzheimer's Disease and Frontotemporal Dementia (Gene) Mutations website. Below is a synopsis of these 7 groups.

The scientific naming (nomenclature) is done in the following manner. Example: R406W tauopathy — "R" is for the protein, arginine, "406" is for the site on the Microtubular Associated Protein Tau gene (Mapt), and "W" is for tryptophane protein.

1. **Amyloid Precursor Proteins (APP) – located on Chromosome 21.**
   Beta - Amyloid is found in the brain tissue of Alzheimer's patients. There are 36 faulty gene mutations of amyloid. This protein is almost always found in the inheritable forms of Alzheimer's disease.

2. **Presenilin I (PSEN 1) – located on Chromosome 14.**
   This group of proteins is known to cause the early-onset form of Alzheimer's disease. There are 182 faulty gene mutations of Presenilin I.

3. **Presenilin II (PSEN II) – located on Chromosome 1.**
   PSEN I and 2 are predominately found in the Endo-plasmic reticulum and a Golgi complex in the cytoplasm of the cell. There are 23 Presenilin II faulty genes. These proteins play a significant roll in early-onset Alzheimer's disease.

4. **Tau Proteins, also designated as Microtubular Associated Protein Tau (MAPT) – Gene errors are located on Chromosome 17.**
   There are 6 configurations of Tau, 3 of which are normal, and 3 are abnormal (hyper-phosphorylated). There are 66 Tau (MAPT) Mutations.

5. **Transcription-activated DNA binding Proteins (TARDBP)**
   TARDBP is also known as **TDP-43**. This group of faulty proteins is also referred to as "Progranulin" proteins. It is associated with wound repair. **This error in protein is located on Chromosome 1** and is found in Frontotemporal Lobar Dementia (FTLD) and motor neuron diseases (Lou Gehrig's disease). There are 123 faulty TARDBP (progranulin) (TDP-43) genes.

6. **Chromatin Modifying Proteins (CHMP2B) – Gene mutation on Chromosome 3.** This faulty gene has been described in a single family in Denmark. There are 10 gene faults of CHMP2B.

7. **Vasoline Containing Protein (VCP).**

The Brain

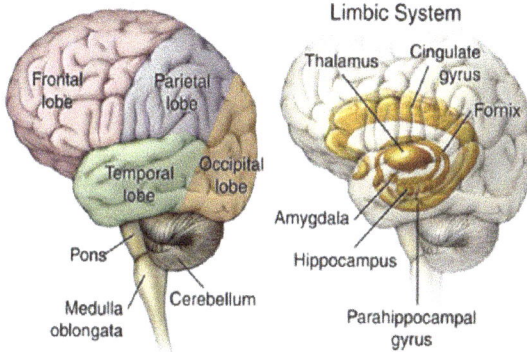

Limbic System

The left view is the outside of the brain, showing frontal, parietal, temporal, occipital lobes and the brain stem structures.

On the right is a view of the internal structures of the brain.

Listed below is a glossary of terms pictured here and needed to understand a discussion of how the brain is changed in these dementias.

© 2000 - 2010 American Health Assistance Foundation

Glossary of Terms for an Anatomy of the Brain

Amygdala – limbic structure involved in many brain functions, including emotion, learning and memory. It is part of a system that processes "reflexive" emotions like fear and anxiety.

Cerebellum – governs movement.

Cingulate gyrus – plays a role in processing conscious emotional experience.

Fornix – an arch-like structure that connects the hippocampus to other parts of the limbic system.

Frontal lobe – helps control skilled muscle movements, mood, planning for the future, setting goals and judging priorities.

Hippocampus – plays a significant role in the formation of long-term memories.

Medulla oblongata – contains centers for the control of vital processes such as heart rate, respiration, blood pressure, and swallowing.

Limbic system – a group of interconnected structures that mediate emotions, learning, and memory.

Occipital lobe – helps process visual information.

Parahippocampal gyrus – an important connecting pathway of the limbic system.

Parietal lobe – receives and processes information about temperature, taste, touch, and movement coming from the rest of the body. Reading and arithmetic are also processed in this region.

Pons – contains centers for the control of vital processes, including respiration and cardiovascular functions. It also is involved in the coordination of eye movements and balance.

Temporal lobe – processes hearing, memory and language functions.

Thalamus – a major relay station between the senses and the cortex (the outer layer of the brain consisting of the parietal, occipital, frontal and temporal lobes).

From observing the diagram above, one can note that it is the frontal and temporal lobes of the brain that are affected initially by the FTLD dementias. It is the parietal lobe that is initially and primarily affected in Alzheimer's Disease. Being that both these diseases are progressive, eventually the entire brain is diseased.

Cross section of a Normal and a Diseased Brain From Front View

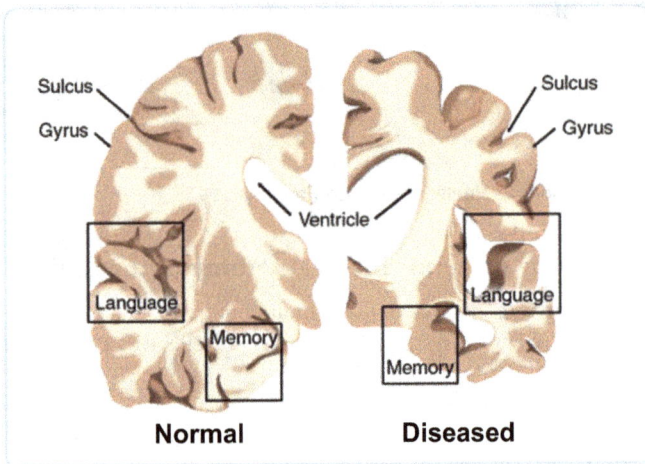

© 2000 - 2010 American Health Assistance Foundation

In Alzheimer's disease, there is an overall shrinkage of brain tissue, the sulci (plural of sulcus) are noticeably widened, and there is shrinkage of the gyri (plural of gyrus). In addition, the ventricles within the brain are noticeably enlarged. In the early stages of Alzheimer's disease and some forms of FTLD, short-term memory begins to fade when the cells in the hippocampus degenerate. Activities of daily living become difficult. Judgment declines, emotional outbursts may occur, and language is impaired as dementia spreads. As more nerve cells die, changes in behavior, such as wandering and agitation occurs. Their ability to recognize faces and to communicate deteriorates in the final stages, and the patient at this stage requires constant care.

The complexity of the human brain is evident by the fact that it contains approximately 50 to 100 billion neurons. Each of those neurons has 10,000 synaptic connections to other neurons. Roughly one billion synapses are present in each cubic millimeter of cerebral cortex. These neurons communicate with one another by means of synapse of the axons, which carry information to other parts of the brain or body. Below is a diagram of the structure of the Neuron and a glossary of terms.

Microscopic Structure of a Neuron

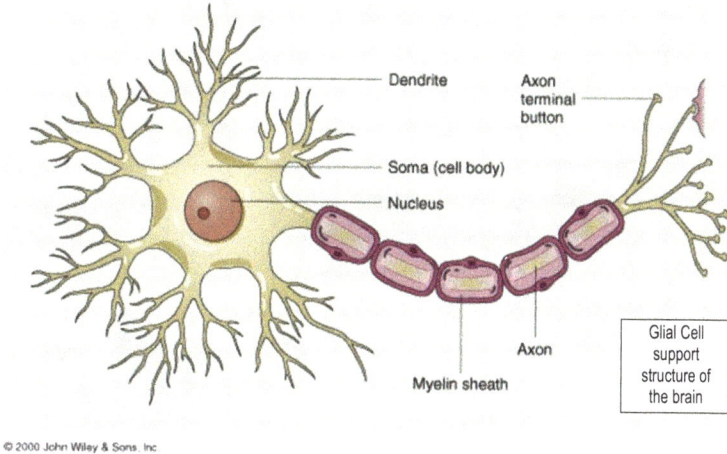

© 2000 John Wiley & Sons, Inc.

Glossary of Terms for the Structure of a Neuron

axon – the long extension of a neuron that carries nerve impulses away from the body of the cell.

axon terminals – the hair-like ends of the axon

cell body (soma) – the cell body of the neuron; it contains the nucleus (also called the soma)

dendrites – the branching structure of a neuron that receives messages (attached to the cell body)

myelin sheath – the fatty substance that surrounds and protects some nerve fibers

nucleus – the organelle in the cell body of the neuron that contains the genetic material of the cell

80% of the brain is made up of glial cells that act as the structure of the brain. 20% of the brain is made up of 50- to 100-billion neurons.

In the diagram above, the neurofibrillary tangles would be in the soma (cell body) of the neurons. The amyloid plaques would be found among the glial cell support structure. It is believed that the amyloid plaques and the neurofibrillary tangles cause brain death. ❖

Chapter 11

Advance Planning

Long Term Care Disability Insurance
Your lifeline to the future

L ong Term Care insurance is not just insurance for the elderly. It is insurance to provide monetary help for any individual who can no longer work. There are a multitude of ways young people become disabled and need long term care insurance. Automobile, industrial, and leisure accidents, Multiple Sclerosis, early-onset Alzheimer's disease, and FTLDs are just a few of the reasons living expenses and assets may need to be protected.

Purchase Long Term Care (LTC) from a reputable company, an agent you can trust, and in an amount you can afford, even a bit more than you think you can afford.

For most people, LTC Insurance is a question of affordability. What is the least amount I can get by with, and how do I pay for what I need? LTC is more affordable if purchased early in life. Unfortunately, 80% of new purchasers are already in their 60s or beyond, and it is very expensive to purchase at that age.

It is very hard to rationalize purchasing LTC Insurance early in life when the family has the most number of expenses. Some of those expenses include the cost of daily living (food, housing, heating, clothing), preparing to send children to college, preparing for retirement, and with the "sandwich" generation, helping the parents with aging issues and expenses. Most people rationalize that they should buy as little as they can afford. Later, when financial help is needed, the purchaser looks back and wishes they had tried to find a way to purchase a larger policy. It would appear to be reasonable to buy just enough to protect the future, "just in case we need it." After all "insurance" is about spreading the risk.

As with the other issues of health care, understanding the insurance language is almost impossible without a guide. If you obtain five LTC policies to review, even the language between the five, is confusing. You must find a guide, an agent who specializes in LTC to help you. Select a nationally-known company, and check to see if they are financially healthy. It would be a shame to pay LTC premiums for 25 years and then, when you need the care, to find that the company you selected has gone under, leaving you with no coverage after paying premiums for all of those years. In the past, many employers offered LTC insurance as part of their "benefits" package. In these difficult financial times, however, many of these companies are eliminating this benefit.

Many states have an agency called **The Assurance Association** that will pay the benefits being charged by a qualified institution **if the insured is already receiving benefits** when the Insurance company goes out of business. The state Assurance Association will only pay up to a certain amount; for example, $350,000 over the lifetime of the insured. If individuals have not started receiving benefits when the company goes under, there is no safety net. The premiums paid are lost, and no benefits will be paid out by the Insurance Company or Assurance Association.

How does an individual decide what they can afford and how to purchase LTC? As with buying anything, the more you buy, the more expensive it becomes.

What follows is a "Reader's Digest" version of what you should know.

LTC has three types of coverage and comes as a package. You get all three types of coverage when you make your purchase. The three coverages are:
1. Home care
2. Assisted Living care
3. Convalescent care.

A **premium** is your monthly/quarterly/annual payment for coverage. A **benefit** is what the insurance company will pay the provider of the service. Home care and Assisted Living benefits are usually one-half of the Convalescent care benefits. If the company offers a **Lifetime benefit**, the value may be for a specific time or number of dollars, i.e., seven years or

$350,000. For some caregivers, this amount may be insufficient. The Insurance Company needs to state, **Lifetime UNLIMITED Benefits**. The numbers of insurance companies providing this level of benefit will become more difficult to find for those victims of FTLDs, Early-onset Alzheimer's, and some others diseases. Lifetime UNLIMITED Benefits are the only reasonable choice, if available.

Example: If one selects $150.00 per day benefit for Convalescent Care, the maximal benefit for Home Care and Assisted Living is $75.00 per day. Home Care, Assisted Living and Convalescent Care can be perceived as three different contracts. Even if the benefit from Home Care is used up, when your loved one is needing Assisted Living, the Insurance will then again be available for them to a certain amount. Likewise, when Convalescent Care is needed, that benefit goes into effect.

How do you calculate what protection you need or want (which may not be what you can afford)? Call three to five Convalescent Care facilities that you feel would provide the care to your loved one that is acceptable to you. Ask the business department their average COST of daily care (or monthly). If they tell you $5,000 per month, that means it is $165 per day.

As you review the five responses, assume the most expensive response is the one you wish to accept as the "daily" benefit for your insurance policy.

In actuality, you could accept this as your only benefit. But … there are other coverage benefits called "Riders" that the insurance companies can add to your policy.

One kind of Rider you should want to accept is an "Inflation" Rider. We all know the cost of health care services is increasing at a rate higher than almost any other industry. If the potential use of the LTC insurance benefits are years into the future, it would be wise to choose this Rider.

An additional Rider is called a "Waiver of Premium." This Rider allows the payer of the premium to NOT pay the premium after the insured has begun to a receive benefits. There is usually a 90-day (3 month) wait period where you continue to pay premiums. After this 90 days, all premiums are waived (not paid) anymore.

The purchaser of LTC insurance is caught in a quandary. They may desperately need to add these Riders but cannot afford the increase to the premium. Please discuss this with your financial consultant or other social services agencies for other methods of meeting this financial need.

Assisted Living Admissions
by Francis Coates
Director of Margorie McCune Center
North Carolina

What is Assisted Living
Sometimes referred to as "domiciliary care" or "rest homes"

Assisted Living provides care to the elderly and disabled in an environment of "choices," offering individuals as much freedom, independence, privacy and dignity as possible while providing service of basic human needs such as medication administration, bathing, meals, housekeeping, shopping, transportation, outings, socialization and events. The individualized care plan is monitored by an RN.

Unlike a nursing home, assisted living care is mainly provided by unlicensed nursing staff. Professionals such as physicians, podiatrists, psychiatrists, psychologists, therapists, and nutritionists, are contracted for weekly visits or less. Transportation is provided for medical appointments, dentists, specialists, etc. Other staff such as dietary, activity director, and housekeeping generally have to meet the same requirements of nursing homes. Assisted living is for the individuals who are looking for services for activities of daily living (ADL) but don't require the intensive medical skills that nursing homes provide.

Qualifications for Admission

Typically, families or hospital caseworkers initiate the original contact for an individual to seek assisted living. Family members or caseworkers notice varying degrees of either physical or mental health limitations. The individual exhibits behaviors that present a reasonable likelihood of serious harm to self or others, such as leaving stove burners on, over or under medication administration, the need for assistance in meal preparation, ambulation, chronic memory loss, loss of bladder and bowel control, acute weight gain or loss, unsanitary or unsafe housekeeping practices, inability to transport themselves, amongst other possible indicators that the individual is no longer able to care safely for themselves.

The possible need for care is addressed with the individual's physician. If the physician determines the need for care, he/she will initiate a form called an FL2 (North Carolina requirement). The FL2 lists the individual's level of care needs. One category is Domiciliary. At this point the 'decision maker' can determine if this is the best course of action for the individual. Often the 'decision maker' is the individual themselves. If determined that the doctor's determination is that the individual qualifies for Domiciliary care; that individual now qualifies for assisted living. An assisted living center cannot admit an individual without the FL2 [in North Carolina]. The center will also need a Diet Order from the physician and a current TB test result.

DSS can provide a listing of assisted living facilities in the area. The Internet also provides this information for all areas on many different sites. A rating system also went into affect in 2009 that is called the "Four Star Rating System." The first year, this new rating allowed only three stars maximum. The full four stars are now available. This determination is based on an annual survey provided by the state. There are other resources available to find the success of a center. The health department surveys and grades centers on a quarterly basis. The DSS does monthly monitoring of all assisted living centers that accept Medicaid funding.

However, the best way to assess a center to determine if it's best for you is to spend some time in the center. Watch the interactions of the staff with the residents of the center, look at the staff turnover, the staff and resident ratio. Interview the residents of the center, "Are you happy here? What is it like to live at this center?" Taste, smell, and watch the service of the food. Are the residents active or sitting listlessly for long periods of time? Do the residents interact with one another, or seem detached? Check to see if the center meets your individual requirements. If you need a center that allows a smoking area, you don't want to move into one that has strict no smoking policies. If privacy is important to you, but all that the center offers is a semi-private room, you will be less satisfied than if you could have a private room without a shared bathroom. It's very important to know that your individual dignity and rights will be respected.

Another factor is the center's retention policy. If ambulation is your individual concern and the center discharges residents who require a walker, wheelchair, or scooter and this will soon be a necessity for your individual needs, be aware that you may have to move soon.

The assisted living center will then provide you with information, a tour, and an admission packet to fill out. Again, read the packet closely. It will ask questions as to who opens your mail, where your money goes and who handles it, and it will provide you with the center's policies and additional costs, amongst other things.

Finances and Insurances

Many assisted living centers are private pay only. Long-term care insurance, when set up correctly, is an excellent resource. A well written policy can pay the assisted living costs and percentages of other costs, such as ambulance, medications, etc. Be aware that many of the long-term care insurance policies do not cover care in an assisted living facility unless you specify coverage. Terms to look out for are "Only covers skilled care." Typically, the consumer thinks that is all nursing centers. What this term means is "Only covers nursing homes." In 1999, the most common basic price range was between $12,000 and $24,000 per year. In most Assisted Living Centers, this cost does not cover all services. The residents pay extra for such essentials as medications, physicians, dentists, specialists, ambulances, clothing, beauticians, restaurants, events, gifts at holidays, their automobiles, etc., depending upon their individual needs. Private pay monies usually come from the individual residents' retirement monies, social security checks, and/or assistance from families, pensions, etc.

North Carolina has incorporated assisted living money availability into the Medicaid program. This has been a great benefit to many seniors and disabled individuals. According to data from the U.S. Census Bureau, 40 percent of persons aged 75 and older had incomes in 1997 of less than $10,000 per year. Eighty-four percent of persons aged 75 and older had incomes of less than $25,000 per year in 1997, making assisted living unaffordable for the vast majority of older persons. Medicaid allows a person who receives under $1,200.00 per month and has a savings of $2,000 or less to receive assistance that permits them access to an assisted living center, even if they own a home. ❖

Appendix

*O*n the following pages, we are showing examples of legal documents that you will need to acquire, fill out, have notarized, and have filed with your county courthouse should you be faced with the long-term care of a loved one. The forms shown here are, of course, from the author's home state of North Carolina. You will need to acquire legal forms from your own home state. Many of the blank forms can be downloaded from the Internet.

The forms we suggest that you fill out and have filed are:

- A Living Will
- A Power of Attorney for both financial and health care
- A Personal Will for each of you
- Medicaid Long Term Care Services

These Sample Documents are NOT to be COPIED or USED as Legal Documents.

All Samples of Documents found on the following pages are for your Evaluation Only.

LIVING WILL

LIVING WILL
And
HEALTH CARE POWER-OF-ATTORNEY

1. **DESIGNATION OF HEALTH CARE AGENT.**

I, ___NAME___, BEING OF SOUND MIND, HEREBY APPOINT:

NAME:
HOME ADDRESS:
HOME TELEPHONE NUMBER:
WORK TELEPHONE NUMBER:

As my health care Attorney-in-fact (herein referred to as my ("health care agent") to act for me and in my name (in any way I could act in person) to make health care decisions for me as authorized in this document.

2. **EFFECTIVENESS OF APPOINTMENT.**

Absent revocation, the authority granted in this document shall become effective when and if the physician or physicians designated below determine that I lack sufficient understanding or capacity to make or communicate decisions relating to my health care and will continue in effect during my following physician or physicians.

NAME:
ADDRESS:
TELEPHONE NUMBER

NAME:
ADDRESS:
TELEPHONE NUMBER

3. **GENERAL STATEMENT OF AUTHORITY GRANTED.**

EXCEPT as indicated in Section 4 below, I hereby grant to my health care agent named above full power and authority to make health care decisions on my behalf, including, but not limited to, the following:

- To request, review, and receive any information, verbal or written, regarding my physical or mental health, including, but not limited to, medical and hospital records, and to consent to the disclosure of this information;

- To employ or discharge my health care providers;

- To consent to and authorize my admission to and discharge from a hospital, nursing or convalescent home, or other institution;

Figure 1: Living Will and Health Care Power-of-Attorney, page 1

- To give consent for, to withdraw consent for, or to withhold consent for, X-ray, anesthesia, medication, surgery, and all other diagnostic and treatment procedures ordered by or under the authorization of a licensed physician, dentist, or podiatrist. This authorization specifically includes the power to consent to measures for relief of pain.

- To authorize the withholding or withdrawal of life-sustaining procedures when and if my physician determines that I am terminally ill, permanently in a coma, suffer severe dementia, or am in a persistent vegetative state. Life-sustaining procedures are those forms of medical care that only serve to artificially prolong the dying process and may include mechanical ventilation, dialysis, antibiotics, artificial nutrition and hydration, and other forms of medical treatment which sustain, restore or supplant vital bodily functions. Life sustaining procedures do not include care necessary to provide comfort or alleviate pain.

> **I DESIRE THAT MY LIFE NOT BE PROLONGED BY LIFE-SUSTAINING PROCEDURES IF I AM TERMINALLY ILL, PERMANENTLY IN A COMA, SUFFER SEVERE DEMENTIA, OR AM IN A PERSISTENT VEGETATIVE STATE.**

- To exercise any right I may have to make a disposition of any part or all of my body for medical purposes, to donate my organs, to authorize an autopsy, and to direct the disposition of my remains.

- To make any lawful actions that may be necessary to carry out these decisions, including the granting of releases of liability to medical providers.

4. **SPECIAL PROVISIONS AND LIMITATIONS**.

> In exercising the authority to make health care decisions on my behalf, the authority of my health care agent is subject to the following special provisions and limitations.

5. **GUARDIANSHIP PROVISION**.

> If it becomes necessary for a court to appoint a guardian of my person, I nominate my health care agent acting under this document to be the guardian of my person, to serve without bond or security.

6. **RELIANCE OF THIRD PARTIES ON HEALTH CARE AGENT**.

   o No person who relies in good faith upon the authority of any representations by my health care agent shall be liable to me, my estate, my heirs, successors, assigns, or personal representative, for actions or omissions by my health care agent.

   o The powers conferred on my health care agent by this document may be exercised by my health care agent alone, and my health care agent's signature or act under the authority granted in this document my be accepted by persons as fully authorized by me and with the same force and effect as if I were personally present, competent, and acting on my own behalf. All acts performed in good faith by my health care agent pursuant to this Power-of-Attorney are done with my consent and shall have the same validity and effect as if I were present and exercised the powers myself and shall inure to the benefit of and

Figure 2: Living Will and Health Care Power-of-Attorney, page 2

bind me, my estate, my heirs, successors, assigns, and personal representatives. The authority of my health care agent pursuant to this Power-of-Attorney shall be superior to and binding upon my family, relatives, friends, and others.

7. **MISCELLANEOUS PROVISIONS:**

o I revoke any prior Health Care Power-of-Attorney.

o My health care agent shall be entitled to sign, execute, deliver and acknowledge any contract or other document that may be necessary, desirable, convenient, or proper in order to exercise and carry out any of the powers described in this document and to incur reasonable costs on my behalf incident to the exercise of these powers; provided, however, that except as shall be necessary in order to exercise the powers described in this document relating to my health care agent shall not have any authority over my property or financial affairs.

o My health care agent and my health care agent's estate, heirs, successors, and assigns are hereby released and forever discharged by me, my estate, my heirs, successors, assigns, and personal representatives from all liability and from all claims or demands of all kinds arising out of the acts or omissions of my health care agent pursuant to this document, except for willful misconduct or gross negligence.

o No act or omission by my health care agent, or of any other person, institution, or facility acting in good faith in reliance on the authority of my health care agent pursuant to this health care power of attorney shall be considered suicide, nor the cause of my death for any civil or criminal purposes, nor shall it be considered unprofessional conduct or as lack of professional competence. Any person, institution, or facility against whom criminal or civil liability is asserted because of conduct authorized by this health care power-of-attorney may interpose this document as a defense.

8. **SIGNATURE OF PRINCIPAL**.

By signing here, I indicate that I am mentally alert and competent, fully informed as to the contents of this document, and understand the full import of this grant of powers to my health care agent.

This the _____ day of _____, 2010.

_____(SEAL)

9. **SIGNATURE OF WITNESSES**.

I hereby state that the Principal, _____, being of sound mind, signed the foregoing Health Care Power-of-Attorney in my presence, and that I am not related to the principal by blood or marriage, and I would not be entitled to any portion of the estate of the principal under any existing will or codicil of the principal or as an heir under the Interstate Succession Act, if the principal died on this date without a Will. I also state that I am not the principal's attending physician, nor any employee of the principal's attending physician, nor an employee of the health facility in which the

Figure 3: Living Will and Health Care Power-of-Attorney, page 3

principal is a patient, nor any employee of a nursing home or any group care home where the principal resides. I further state that I do not have any claim against the principal.

This the _____ day of _____, 2010.

_____
WITNESS

_____
WITNESS

STATE OF NORTH CAROLINA

COUNTY OF

C E R T I F I C A T E

    I, the undersigned Notary Public for the County and State aforesaid, hereby certify that ___NAME_____, appeared before me and swore to me and to the witnesses in my presence that this instrument is a Health Care Power-of-Attorney and that she willingly and voluntarily made and executed it as her free act and deed for the purposes expressed in it.

    I further certify that ___name of witness_____ and ___name of witness_____, witnessed, appeared before me and swore that they witnessed him/her sign the attached Health Care Power-of-Attorney, believing him/her to be of sound mind; and also swore that at the time they witnessed the signing (i) they were not related within the third degree to him/her or him/her spouse, and (ii) they did not know nor have a reasonable purpose for not signing this document.

_____
Notary Public

Figure 4: Living Will and Health Care Power-of-Attorney, page 4

POWER OF ATTORNEY

KNOW ALL MEN BY THESE PRESENTS:

THAT I, _____, a legal resident of the State of North

Carolina, do hereby **revoke** and declare null and void any Power-of-Attorney which I

have heretofore executed and by these presents do make, constitute and appoint

_____, my true and lawful Attorney-in-Fact to act, manage and

conduct all of my estate and all of my affairs and for that purpose for me and in my

name, place and stead, and for my use and benefit and as my act and deed, to do and

execute, or to concur with persons, jointly interested with myself, therein in the doing or

executing of all or any of the following acts, deeds and things as such may be defined in

Chapter 32A of the North Carolina General Statutes to the extent that I am permitted by

law to act through an agent:

1. To buy, receive, lease, accept or otherwise acquire, to sell, convey, mortgage, hypothecate, pledge, quitclaim or otherwise encumber or dispose of, or to contract or agree for the acquisition, disposal or the encumbrance of any property whatsoever and wheresoever situated, be it real, personal or mixed, or any custody, possession, interest or right therein, or pertaining thereto, upon such terms as my said Attorney shall think proper.

2. To take, hold, possess, invest, lease or let or otherwise manage any or all of my real, personal or mixed property, or any right or interest therein or pertaining thereto; to eject, remove or relieve tenants or other persons from and recover possession of such property by all lawful means and to maintain, protect, preserve, insure, remove, store, transport, repair, rebuild, modify or improve the same or any part thereof.

3. To make, do and transact business of whatever kind or nature, including the receipt, recovery, collection, payment, compromise, settlement, endorsement, negotiation and adjustment of all accounts, legacies, bequests, interests, dividends, annuities, claims, U.S. Government bonds, Government securities, demands, debts, taxes and obligations, which may now or hereafter be due, owing or payable by me or to me.

4. To make, endorse, accept, receive, sign, seal, acknowledge, execute and deliver deeds, assignments, agreements, certificates, hypothecations, checks, notes, bonds, vouchers, receipts, releases and such other instruments in writing or whatsoever kind and nature as may be necessary.

Figure 5: Power-of-Attorney, page 1

5. To ask, demand, sue for, recover, collect and receive each and every sum of money, debt, account, legacy, bequest, interest, dividend, annuity and demand (which now is or hereafter shall become due, owing and payable) belonging to or claimed by me, and to use and take any lawful means for the recovery thereof by legal process or otherwise, and to execute and deliver a satisfaction or release therefore, together with the right and power to compromise or compound any claim or demand.

6. To make deposits or investments in, or withdrawals from, any account, holding or interest which I may now or hereafter have or be entitled to in any baking, trust or investment institution, including postal savings, depository offices, credit unions, savings and loan associations and similar institutions; to exercise any right, option or privilege pertaining thereto, and to open or establish accounts, holdings or interests of whatsoever kind or nature with any institution in my name or in my said Attorney's name or in our names jointly, either with or without right-of-survivorship.

7. To contract loans and to borrow any sums of money in my name and upon such terms as my said Attorney shall see fit and to pledge or give as security therefore any or all of my property. Should such loans be guaranteed to any lender under the provisions of any laws of the United States or any State, my said Attorney is authorized to sign on my behalf any and all documents or instruments required by such laws or governmental agencies.

8. To act as my Attorney or proxy in respect to any bonds, stocks, shares, life insurance or other investments, rights, options or interests I now or hereafter hold, excluding however, in the case of life insurance, the right to change the method of payment of the insurance proceeds and the right to make a cash surrender of the policy as distinguished from the surrender of the policy for loan, conversion or other purposes as provided herein.

9. To occupy, expend or use all or any part of my estate as now or hereafter constituted for the care, support maintenance and benefit of me.

10. To engage and dismiss agents, counsel and employees and to appoint and remove at pleasure any substitute for, or agent of, my said Attorney in respect to all or any of the matters or things herein mentioned.

11. To prepare, execute and file income and other tax returns, any governmental reports, declarations, applications, requests and documents.

12. To have access to any safe deposit box or boxes that may be now or hereafter rented by me, or standing in my name; to withdraw or remove any of the contents thereof and to make deposits in and otherwise use or surrender such box or boxes; and to rent any safe deposit box or boxes in my name, or in my said Attorney's name or in our names jointly, either with or without right-of-survivorship.

13. To extend and renew all notes and liens executed by me or by my said Attorney-in-Fact upon such terms and conditions as she may deem proper.

14. The Power-of-Attorney is to continue in effect and shall not be affected by my subsequent incapacity or mental incompetence, pursuant to Chapter 32A of the General Statutes of North Carolina and amendments thereto, until my death or until I revoke this Power-of-Attorney in writing.

Figure 6: Power-of-Attorney, page 2

N WITNESS WHEREOF, I have hereunto set my hand and seal, this the _____ day of
_____, 2010.

                               _____(SEAL)
                                          Name

****

NORTH CAROLINA

_____ COUNTY

      On the _____ day of _____, 2010, personally appeared before me, the said
named _____, to me known and known to me to be the person described in
and who executed the foregoing instrument and he acknowledged that he executed the same
and being duly sworn by me, made oath that the statements in the foregoing instrument are
true.

      My commission expires: _____

                                 _____
                                      Notary Public

Figure 7: Power-of-Attorney, page 3

WILL

I, _____, of _____ County, North Carolina, declare this to be my Last Will, hereby revoking all Wills and Codicils heretofore made by me.

ARTICLE I

I direct that all my just debts, funeral expenses including the cost of a suitable monument at my grave and the costs of the administration of my estate by paid out of the assets of my estate as soon as practicable after my death.

ARTICLE II

I direct that all estate and inheritance taxes and other taxes in the general nature thereof which shall become payable upon or by reason of my death with respect to any property passing by or under the terms of this Will or any Codicil to it hereafter executed by me, or with respect to the proceeds of any policy or policies of insurance on my life, or with respect to any other property included in my gross estate for the purpose of such taxes, shall be paid by my personal representative out of the principal of my residuary estate, and I direct that no part of any such taxes be charged against (or collected from) the person receiving or in possession of the property taxed, or receiving the benefit thereof, it being my intention that all such persons, legatees, devisee, surviving tenant by the entirety, and beneficiaries receive full benefits without any diminution on account of such taxes.

ARTICLE III

After carrying out the provisions contained above, I give, will and devise all the rest and residue of the property which I may own at the time of death, real and personal, tangible and intangible, of whatsoever nature and wheresoever situated, including all property which I may acquire or become entitled to after the execution of this Will unto my husband/wife, _____, in fee simple, if he is living at my death.

ARTICLE IV

Should my husband/wife predecease me, then after carrying out the provisions contained above, I give, will and device:
The sum of _____ to _____.
Unto _____, etc. etc.

ARTICLE V

Should my husband/wife, _____ predecease me, then after carrying out the provisions contained above, I give, will, and devise all the rest and residue of the property which I may own at the time of my death, real and personal, tangible and intangible, of whatsoever nature and wheresoever situated, including all property which I may acquire or become entitled to after the execution of this Will unto _____, **In Trust**, for my __son/daughter___, __name____, until she shall reach the age of twenty-five (25) years. Etc etc.

Figure 8: Will, page 1

In addition to those powers hereinafter granted to my said Trustee in Article VIII, and not by way of limitation, I hereby grant unto my said Trustee, the right and power, to disburse from principal and/or income such sums as my said Trustee shall, in her sole discretion, deem necessary or appropriate for the use, benefit, health, education, and maintenance of said beneficiary. My Trustee shall not be held liable or answerable for any errors in judgment in making any such distribution.

ARTICLE VI

After carrying out the provisions contained above, should both my husband/wife, _____, and my son/daughter/other relative, predecease me or should we die as a result of a common disaster, I then give, will and devise all the rest and residue of the property which I may own at the time of my death, real and personal, tangible and intangible, of whatsoever nature and wheresoever situated, including all property which I may acquire or become entitled to after the execution of this Will unto _____ etc.etc. I hereby grant unto my said Trustee, or successor Trustee, the right and power, to disburse from principal and/or income such sums as my said Trustee shall, in her sole discretion, deem necessary or appropriate for the use, benefit, health, education, and maintenance of said beneficiary. My Trustee shall not be held liable or answerable for any errors in judgment in making any such distribution.

Upon the death of my Trustee, _____, all assets then constituting said Trust are hereby devised in fee simple unto the Trustees of _____.
This fund shall be used by the Trustees of _____ for the following purposes: Outline your wishes)

ARTICLE VII

Should my husband/wife and I die in a manner that it cannot be determined which of us survived, then it shall be presumed that he/she survived me, and my estate shall be administered and distributed in all respects in accordance with such presumption.

ARTICLE VIII

I appoint my husband/wife, _____, the personal representative of his my Last Will and direct that no surety or other bond be required of my said personal representative.
If my said husband/wife, _____, shall predecease me, or for any reason fail to qualify as my personal representative hereunder, or having qualified shall die or resign, then in that event, I appoint _____ the personal representative and she/he shall have, possess and exercise all powers and authority herein conferred on my original personal representative.
Without in any way limiting the generality of the foregoing and subject to North Carolina General Statutes §32-26, I hereby grant unto my personal representatives all powers set forth in North Carolina General Statutes §32-27, and any amendments thereto, and these powers are incorporated herein by reference and made a part of this instrument and such powers are in addition to and not a substitution of the powers conferred by law, except General Statutes §32-27(29), 28A-13-3(b)(c), 28A-13-3(a)(18), and 28A013-3(a)(20) which expressly shall not apply to my personal representatives or Trustee named herein.

Figure 9: Will, page 2

I, _____, the Testatrix, sign my name to this instrument, this _____ day of _____, and being first duly sworn, do hereby declare to the undersigned authority that I sign and execute this instrument as my Last Will and that I sign it willingly, that I execute it as my free and voluntary act for the purposes therein expressed, and that I am 18 years of age, or older, of sound mind and under no constraint or undue influence.

_____(seal)

We, the undersigned witnesses, sign our names to this instrument, being first duly sworn, and hereby declare to the undersigned authority that _____ signs and executes this instrument as her Last Will and that she signs it willingly and that each of us in the presence and hearing of the Testatrix hereby sign this Will as witnesses to the Testatrix's signing and to the best of our knowledge, Testatrix is 18 years of age, or older, of sound mind and under no constraint or undue influence.

_____
WITNESS

_____
WITNESS

NORTH CAROLINA

_____ COUNTY

Subscribed, sworn to and acknowledge before me by _____, the Testatrix, and subscribed and sworn to before me by _____ and _____, witnesses, this _____ day of _____, 2010.

_____
Notary Public

My commission expires: _____

Figure 10: Will, page 3

FL-2 (86)
INSTRUCTIONS ON REVERSE SIDE

NORTH CAROLINA MEDICAID PROGRAM
LONG TERM CARE SERVICES

☐ PRIOR APPROVAL   ☐ UTILIZATION REVIEW   ☐ ON-SITE REVIEW

IDENTIFICATION

1. PATIENT'S LAST NAME   FIRST   MIDDLE | 2. BIRTHDATE (M/D/Y) | 3. SEX | 4. ADMISSION DATE (CURRENT LOCATION)

5. COUNTY AND MEDICAID NUMBER | 6. FACILITY   ADDRESS | 7. PROVIDER NUMBER

8. ATTENDING PHYSICIAN NAME AND ADDRESS | 9. RELATIVE NAME AND ADDRESS

10. CURRENT LEVEL OF CARE
___ HOME   ___ DOMICILIARY
___ SNF   (REST HOME)
___ ICF   ___ OTHER
___ HOSPITAL

11. RECOMMENDED LEVEL OF CARE
___ HOME   ___ DOMICILIARY
___ SNF   (REST HOME)
___ ICF   ___ OTHER

12. PRIOR APPROVAL NUMBER

13. DATE APPROVED/DENIED

14. DISCHARGE PLAN
___ SNF   ___ HOME
___ ICF
___ DOMICILIARY (REST HOME)
___ OTHER

15. ADMITTING DIAGNOSES - PRIMARY, SECONDARY, DATES OF ONSET

1.   5.
2.   6.
3.   7.
4.   8.

16. PATIENT INFORMATION

DISORIENTED	AMBULATORY STATUS	BLADDER	BOWEL
CONSTANTLY	AMBULATORY	CONTINENT	CONTINENT
INTERMITTENTLY	SEMI-AMBULATORY	INCONTINENT	INCONTINENT
INAPPROPRIATE BEHAVIOR	NON-AMBULATORY	INDWELLING CATHETER	COLOSTOMY
WANDERER	**FUNCTIONAL LIMITATIONS**	EXTERNAL CATHETER	**RESPIRATION**
VERBALLY ABUSIVE	SIGHT	**COMMUNICATION OF NEEDS**	NORMAL
INJURIOUS TO SELF	HEARING	VERBALLY	TRACHEOSTOMY
INJURIOUS TO OTHERS	SPEECH	NON-VERBALLY	OTHER:
INJURIOUS TO PROPERTY	CONTRACTURES	DOES NOT COMMUNICATE	O2 PRN CONT
OTHER:	**ACTIVITIES/SOCIAL**	**SKIN**	**NUTRITION STATUS**
PERSONAL CARE ASSISTANCE	PASSIVE	NORMAL	DIET
BATHING	ACTIVE	OTHER:	SUPPLEMENTAL
FEEDING	GROUP PARTICIPATION	DECUBITI-DESCRIBE:	SPOON
DRESSING	RE-SOCIALIZATION		PARENTERAL
TOTAL CARE	FAMILY SUPPORTIVE		NASOGASTRIC
PHYSICIAN VISITS	**NEUROLOGICAL**		GASTROSTOMY
30 DAYS	CONVULSIONS/SEIZURES		INTAKE AND OUTPUT
60 DAYS	GRAND MAL	DRESSINGS:	FORCE FLUIDS
OVER 180 DAYS	PETIT MAL		WEIGHT
	FREQUENCY		HEIGHT

17. SPECIAL CARE FACTORS

SPECIAL CARE FACTORS	FREQUENCY	SPECIAL CARE FACTORS	FREQUENCY
BLOOD PRESSURE		BOWEL AND BLADDER PROGRAM	
DIABETIC URINE TESTING		RESTORATIVE FEEDING PROGRAM	
PT (BY LICENSED PT)		SPEECH THERAPY	
RANGE OF MOTION EXERCISES		RESTRAINTS	

18. MEDICATIONS / NAME & STRENGTHS, DOSAGE & ROUTE

1.   7.
2.   8.
3.   9.
4.   10.
5.   11.
6.   12.

19. X RAY AND LABORATORY FINDINGS/DATE:

20. ADDITIONAL INFORMATION:

21. PHYSICIAN'S SIGNATURE | 22. DATE

372-124 (12-92)

Figure 11: Medicaid Program Long Term Care Services

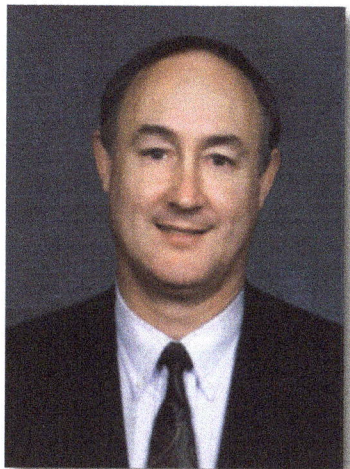

Meet The Author

John H. "Herb" van Roekel

*H*erb van Roekel has had a lifetime passion to be a servant to those in need. Long before he had knowledge that an autosomal dominant gene for R406W tauopathy dementia traveled through the genes of his wife's family, he had made his career serving in the medical arts field in chemistry and clinical laboratory technology. His path led him into medical sales with a large microbiology corporation, and he later became the owner of Navco Supply, Inc. He is currently owner and innkeeper of Raspberry Hill Bed and Breakfast. He is also CEO of Sonshine Mountain Retreat, Inc., a not-for-profit respite care facility that he and his board are developing to aid besieged caregivers. Both are located in the Black Mountain area of North Carolina.

Herb earned his Bachelor of Science from Barton College (formerly Atlantic Christian College) and his Master of Public Health and Administration from the University of North Carolina, Chapel Hill. He has served for 12 years on the Executive Board of Emmanuel College in North Georgia and 22 years on the General Board of Directors. He served for 20 years as a member of his local Lion's Club.

Throughout his years of service, Herb has earned many honors and awards: Distinguished Service Award from Becton Dickinson Research Center and a three-time winner of the Regional Sales Representative of the Year. He is also a recipient of the prestigious Melvin Jones National Award from the Lion's Club International. In addition to his honors and awards, he is owner of two U.S. patents, and he developed a community blood donation program that was augmented with frozen blood technology.

Herb's wife and sister-in-law are presently in assisted living facilities in the Asheville area. He has two grown daughters and two grandchildren.

Herb is available for speaking engagements on the topics of dementia and family care. He can be reached by e-mail at: SlayTheMonster@gmail.com.